Keto Diet Cookbook for Beginners 2021

Lose Fat Faster by Optimizing your Meal Plan, with Healthy and Easy Low Carb Ketogenic Recipes, All with Pictures

Mery L. Davis

Table of Contents

INTRODUCTION

WHAT IS THE KETOGENIC DIET?

The ketogenic diet is a type of low carb diet and is characterized by the fact that the body learns a new way of generating energy through food.

By consuming a lot of healthy fats and very little carbohydrates, the body enters what is known as "ketosis".

In this state, the body burns fat instead of sugar as fuel for cellular energy. Due to the lack of sugar molecules, the liver is forced to convert fatty acids into so-called " ketone bodies ".

And these ketone bodies are anti-inflammatory and can help you lose weight.

A successfully implemented ketogenic diet must meet the following criteria: The liver produces ketone bodies as an alternative fuel to glucose.

WHAT ARE THE BENEFITS OF A KETOGENIC DIET?

A ketogenic diet always aims to bring the body into so-called " ketosis ". In this ketosis, many people experience several advantages over normal "sugar burning".

But what are the benefits and what is the ketogenic diet used for?

Benefits of the ketogenic diet and ketosis

Anti-inflammatory: The ketogenic diet and the resulting ketosis have a strong anti-inflammatory effect. This is believed to lower the risk of degenerative diseases like Alzheimer's and cancer.

Energy-boosting: The state of ketosis supports the cells, especially the brain, to produce more mitochondria. These mitochondria are the energy power plants of your body and ensure that you are awake and focused from morning to night.

Promotes fat burning: The ketogenic diet can help you lose weight quickly and healthily. The ketone bodies ensure long-term satiety and lowering of hunger hormones (such as ghrelin). This means that you will no longer have food cravings and will no longer have to rely on snacks.

Increases concentration: Ketone bodies are an ideal source of energy for the brain. Once the body has adapted to ketosis, the brain can get up to 75% of the energy from ketone bodies. The brain also benefits from the high consumption of healthy fats, since it consists largely of fat and omega 3 fatty acids that support the health of the brain.

Blood sugar lowering: We receive many testimonials in which people with diabetes report significant improvements in their symptoms. When the ketogenic diet is followed properly, insulin and blood sugar levels stabilize. Important: If you suffer from diabetes, you should have this project accompanied by a doctor who has experience with an LCHF diet before switching.

KETOGENIC FOOD LIST

What foods are keto foods? Our clear ketogenic food list shows you the top 15 ketogenic food groups at a glance:

Meat and poultry

Unprocessed meat contains no carbohydrates, making it perfect for a ketogenic diet. Beef, turkey and chicken provide us with protein and B vitamins. Sausage products such as salami, ham and wieners are also okay if they do not contain any sugary additives or starches.

Note: Reach for products from pasture farming, preferably from organic farms. Avoid too much protein: Prefer high-fat parts, such as pork belly or ribeye.

This is allowed: beef, turkey, chicken, pork, deer, duck, veal, goat, goose, lamb, sheep, turkey, wild boar, offal. Also: salami, ham, Viennese.

Low carb vegetables

Low-carbohydrate vegetables are a major source of vitamins and minerals on the ketogenic food list. Water-rich, green (leaf) vegetables and cabbage vegetables play an important role. With the right choice, you can eat up to 900 g of vegetables a day without affecting ketosis.

Note: Eliminate root vegetables and starchy vegetables such as sweet potatoes, which are high in carbohydrates, from your diet.

This is allowed: Green salads, spinach, broccoli, artichoke, asparagus, cucumber, green peppers, pak choi, Brussels sprouts, white cabbage, cauliflower, Chinese cabbage, kale, celeriac, eggplant, leek, mushrooms, zucchini.

Nuts and seeds

In addition to meat and avocado, natural nuts, seeds and seeds are an important source of fat, which provides us with valuable and essential omega-3 fatty acids and omega-6 fatty acids. They also provide a high-quality nutrient package of minerals such as zinc, iron and magnesium as well as B vitamins. Their filling protein content makes them a great ketogenic snack for in between meals.

Note: Nuts also contain some carbohydrates and will affect your carbohydrate balance. Important: Peanuts are not nutting; they belong to the legume family.

This is allowed: almonds, hazelnuts, macadamia nuts, pecans, walnuts, cashews, pine nuts, pistachios, pumpkin seeds, sesame seeds, sunflower seeds, chia seeds, flax seeds, hemp seeds.

Dark chocolate and cocoa powder

A piece (10 g) of dark chocolate with 85% cocoa provides only 2 g of carbohydrates. Baking or making cocoa with unsweetened cocoa powder will not affect the state of your ketosis.

Note: The high cocoa content in chocolates is mandatory. Use unsweetened cocoa powder that does not contain any other additives.

This is allowed: Chocolate from 70% cocoa, unsweetened cocoa powder, cocoa nibs.

fish

Natural fish is also ketogenic and, in addition to healthy omega-3 fatty acids, provides plenty of protein and keeps you full for a long time. The classic tuna with 0 g of carbohydrates is a very popular, ketogenic food.

Note: Here quality counts instead of quantity: Prefer fresh fish, preferably wild caught and eat it twice a week.

This is allowed: tuna, anchovies, perch, cod, eel, flounder, herring, mackerel, salmon, sardines, turbot, trout, pikeperch, carp, pangasius.

Eggs

Chicken eggs hardly contain any carbohydrates and are rich in protein and vitamins such as A, B and K. Their protein has a high biological value. This provides information about the composition of the amino acids in food and how well these can be used by the body. The higher the value, the better the proteins are metabolized.

Note: For ecological reasons, use organic eggs when buying. For vegetarians, organic eggs are a valuable source of protein in a ketogenic diet. As a meat eater, limit your consumption to prefer proteins from meat and fish.

This is allowed: organic free-range chicken eggs.

cheese

The large selection of different types of cheese also remains with a ketogenic diet. You should primarily choose low-carbohydrate or high-fat cheeses such as camembert, parmesan, feta or mozzarella. But cottage cheese is also established in the ketogenic scene and is a popular and low-fat dip or spread.

Note: Cheese also contains some saturated fat and should only be consumed in moderation. Light products and low-fat cheeses are not ketogenic and therefore taboo.

This is allowed: Harz cheese, sheep cheese, Gouda, mozzarella, Brie, Camembert, Gorgonzola, cottage cheese, ricotta, mascarpone.

Fruit and berries

Finding fruit among the ketogenic foods is not easy. Are allowed berries such as strawberries, and blueberries, carbohydrates 8-10 g per 100 g. And don't forget to include the two rather atypical types of fruit in your diet: avocados and olives.

Note: Tropical fruits contain too much fructose and are not suitable as ketogenic foods.

This is allowed: currants, raspberries, strawberries, cantaloupe, cranberries, blueberries, blackberries, papaya, gooseberries, lemons, limes.

Healthy fats and oils

Medium-chain, so-called MCT fats (Medium Chain Triglycerides) are the keto boosters: They mainly consist of the fatty acids caproic acid, caprylic acid, capric acid and lauric acid and are completely and particularly quickly metabolized. Our body breaks them down directly into ketone bodies. You can use coconut oil here, as it contains many of these fatty acids. Cold-pressed olive oil is great for salads and cold dishes. It not only provides healthy fatty acids, but also has an antioxidant effect.

Note: Prefer pure, cold-pressed and high-quality oils and avoid cheap vegetable products that often contain impurities.

This is allowed: coconut oil, olive oil, MCT oil, avocado oil, macadamia oil, walnut oil, sesame oil, ghee, caprylic acid, cocoa butter, lard, palm oil, nut butter.

Drinks such as unsweetened tea and coffee

Drinking plenty is a must to maintain a healthy water balance and replenish electrolytes. In addition to water, unsweetened teas and coffee are also no problem with a ketogenic diet.

Note: Take a look at the list of ingredients and prefer water and naturally flavored drinks such as cucumber water or tea with fresh ginger.

This is allowed: water, carbonated mineral water, unsweetened tea, herbal teas, unsweetened coffee, cucumber water, coconut milk, nut and almond drinks, bulletproof coffee, lemon and lime juice, vegetable and meat broth.

Dairy products

High fat dairy products are also lower in carbohydrates. They provide you with protein and strengthen your teeth and bones with calcium. So that you can get more sugar from fruits and vegetables, limit your dairy product consumption. Therefore, as with eggs, the following applies: Not too much, unless you are eating a ketogenic vegetarian diet.

Note: Choose fresh, high-quality organic products, even ghee or fresh milk directly from the farm are great, high-quality ketogenic foods.

This is allowed: Whole milk, quark, Greek yogurt, natural yoghurt, cream, sour cream, sour cream.

Seafood and animals

In addition to fresh fish, seafood and animals are also suitable as ketogenic foods. Ketarians particularly value crabs and shrimp for their very low carbohydrate content and high nutrient content. Mussels, for example mussels, are slightly higher in carbohydrates (7 g per 100 g).

Note: Seafood and animals add nutrients to your keto diet, but they are relatively expensive ketogenic foods.

This is allowed: shrimp, caviar, clams, crab, lobster, clams, oysters, shrimp, scallops, squid, lobster, crayfish.

Ketogenic baking ingredients: flours and binders

Traditional flours are not ketogenic, but there are plenty of alternatives that also provide healthy nutrients. However, they behave differently when baking than cereal flours. Many conventional binders such as agar-agar or psyllium husks are also keto-friendly.

Note: Do not directly replace flours in recipes 1: 1 with ketogenic alternatives, as they behave differently.

This is allowed: almond flour, coconut flour, desiccated coconut, psyllium husk flour, pumpkin seed flour, guar flour, carob flour, nut and seed flours, potato fibers, gelatine, apple pectin, psyllium husks, agar gelatin, chia seeds.

Ketogenic sweeteners

Many carbohydrate-free substitute sugars allow coffee or yogurt to be sweetened during a ketogenic diet. The fermented glucose erythritol is tooth-friendly and calorie-free, making it a favorite on the ketogenic food list.

Note: Use artificial sweeteners only in small amounts and treat them as ketogenic "stimulants". Warning: very high consumption can cause gas and diarrhea.

This is allowed: erythritol, stevia, xylitol in small quantities.

Spices and herbs

Spices and herbs add variety to every kitchen - including the ketogenic one. Upgrade the limited food selection with high-quality, pure spices and try out new combinations.

Note: Additives, sugar and flavor enhancers that are not ketogenic can hide in spice mixtures in particular. So, check the list of ingredients carefully.

This is allowed: (Sea) salt, pepper, basil, chili powder, curry, cumin, oregano, thyme, rosemary, sage, turmeric, parsley, coriander, cinnamon, nutmeg, cloves, allspice, ginger, cardamom, paprika, dill.

Who is the ketogenic diet suitable for?

- Chronic inflammation
- acne

Suitable - medical or nutritional supervision recommended

- athlete
- Overweight
- diabetes
- Pressure to perform
- epileptic
- dementia

Unsuitable or only under strict medical or nutritional supervision:

- Biliary problems
- Heart disease
- Thyroid problems
- Underweight
- Increased fat levels in the blood

BREAKFAST

Scrambled eggs from the oven

Cooking time: 25 mins
Total time: 35 mins

INGREDIENTS

- 12 medium eggs
- 300 ml of milk
- 50 gr butter or margarine, melted
- salt and pepper to taste

PREPARATION METHOD

1. Preheat the oven to a hundred seventy-five degree. Pour the melted butter right into a 33 cm x 22 cm baking dish. Now take a large bowl and beat the eggs and salt and pepper. Then add the milk grade by grade simultaneously as you're beating the eggs.
2. When all ingredients are well blended, pour the mixture into the oven dish. Bake the egg mixture inside the preheated oven for 10 minutes. Take the ovenproof dish out of the oven and stir the egg mixture well. Then bake for another 10 to fifteen minutes and serve.

NUTRITIONAL VALUES

Serving Size: 1/6
Calories: 236
Fats: 18.0
Carbohydrates: 3.2
Proteins: 14.2

Breakfast muffins with egg and bacon

Cooking time: 30 mins
Total time: 45 mins

INGREDIENTS

- 4 medium eggs
- 4 slices of bacon or bacon
- 4 tsp melted butter
- 1 slice of cheese
- 2 slices of cheese
- 4 paper aluminum muffin cases
- salt and pepper to taste

PREPARATION METHOD

1. Preheat the oven to a hundred seventy-five degrees. Place the bacon slices in a frying pan and fry over medium heat. Bake until the slice is frivolously browned throughout. Then take away the bacon from the pan and wrap the bacon slices inside the muffin instances.
2. Put a teaspoon of melted butter on the bottom of the muffin tin in each mold. Beat the eggs in a bowl and upload salt and pepper to flavor. Now positioned the eggs in the muffin cups.
3. Place the ramekins on a rack and location within the oven. Bake the bacon and egg truffles within the preheated oven for 10 to 15 minutes. When the muffins are nearly done, vicinity the half slice of cheese on the pinnacle of every muffin and bake them in the oven for some greater minutes till the cheese has melted.

NUTRITIONAL VALUES

Serving Size: 1 muffin
Calories: 174
Fats: 14.3
Carbohydrates: 0.3
Proteins: 10.7

Hüttenkase with strawberries

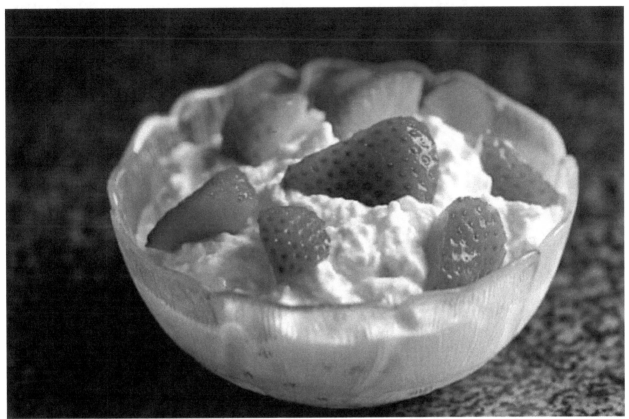

Cooking time: 10 mins   **Total time: 15 mins**

INGREDIENTS

- 170 gr cottage cheese
- 4 small strawberries
- optional: pinch of cinnamon

- optional: grated sugar-free chocolate
- optional: Sweet Bee honey

PREPARATION METHOD

1. Slice the strawberries on a cutting board. Put the cottage cheese in a bowl and add the strawberries to the bowl. To make the recipe even greater delicious, you can sprinkle a bit of cinnamon and grated sugar-unfastened chocolate over the cottage cheese.

NUTRITIONAL VALUES

Serving Size: 1 bowl   0Fats: 6.1   Proteins: 18.0
Calories: 14   Carbohydrates: 6.3

Avocado and green tea powershake

Cooking time: 5 mins　　　　　　　　　　　**Total time: 5 mins**

INGREDIENTS

- 290 ml unsweetened almond milk
- 140 gr Greek yogurt
- 1/2 avocado
- 1/2 scoop vanilla protein powder
- 1 tsp matcha tea powder
- stevia to taste

PREPARATION METHOD

1. Cut the avocado into pieces and positioned the portions inside the blender. Then additionally add the Greek yogurt, protein powder, matcha, and stevia to the blender. Finally, pour the almond milk into the blender. Turn on the blender and blend. Divide the shake between two glasses and enjoy!

NUTRITIONAL VALUES

Serving size: 1 glass　　　　　　Fat: 16.3　　　　　　　　　　Proteins: 11.3

Calories: 230　　　　　　　　　Carbohydrates: 6.0

Paleo breakfast burrito

Cooking time: 10 mins   **Total time: 15 mins**

INGREDIENTS

- 6 thick slices of ham
- 4 medium eggs
- 1/2 onion
- 1/2 red bell pepper
- vegetable of your choice
- salt and pepper to taste

PREPARATION METHOD

2. Cut the onion and bell pepper into small portions on a big cutting board. Then fry the onion in a frying pan over medium warmth. After a couple of baking minutes, add the pepper and fry in short.
3. Then pour the eggs over the greens in the pan. Then grasp a spatula and stir properly to make scrambled eggs.
4. Remove the scrambled eggs with the vegetables from the pan. Divide the scrambled eggs and vegetables over the slices of ham and season with salt and pepper. Then roll the ham tightly, and fry the stuffed ham rolls within the frying pan for some seconds.

NUTRITIONAL VALUES

Serving Size: 1 servings   Fat: 12.5   Proteins: 19.8
Calories: 210   Carbohydrates: 4.1

Protein-rich pancakes

Cooking time: 5 mins   **Total time: 5 mins**

INGREDIENTS

- 1 bag of Dietimeal pancake mix
- 110 ml of cold water or milk
- 1 tbsp butter
- summer fruits to taste

PREPARATION METHOD

1. Pour the contents of a bag right into a bowl. Add one hundred ten ml of cold water or milk and blend till a homogeneous answer. Heat a tablespoon of butter in a frying pan. Pour the pancake mix into the pan and fry the pancake lightly on each facet for 1 to 3 mins.

NUTRITIONAL VALUES

Serving Size: 1 pancake   Fats: 0.2   Proteins: 18.0
Calories: 96   Carbohydrates: 4.1

Mexican scrambled eggs

Cooking time: 10 mins
Total time: 15 mins

INGREDIENTS

- 3 medium eggs
- 30 gr grated cheddar cheese
- 1/2 stalk of spring onion
- 1 - 2 pieces of jalapeños from a jar
- 1/4 onion
- 1/2 Roma tomato
- handful of parsley
- 1 tbsp butter or olive oil
- salt and pepper to taste
- optional: low- carb tortilla

PREPARATION METHOD

1. Cut the spring onions, jalapeños, parsley, and onion into small pieces on a large cutting board. Then take the tomato and cut it into small portions as properly. Place the tomato pieces on a paper towel and drain them in short.
2. Then take a medium bowl and beat the eggs in it. Heat a tablespoon of olive oil in a frying pan and fry the spring onions, onions, and jalapeños. Add the eggs and season with salt and pepper. Let the egg set slowly. As quickly because the egg starts to set at the rims, slide the egg from the threshold to the middle with a spatula and stir the entirety collectively properly.
3. When the scrambled eggs are almost ready, upload the tomato and parsley portions and fry for 1 minute greater. Divide among a plate and garnish with a bit of cheese. Enjoy your meal!

NUTRITIONAL VALUES

Serving Size: 1 portion   Fat: 28.7   Proteins: 21.7
Calories: 365   Carbohydrates: 4.3

Low-carbohydrate almond waffles

Cooking time: 10 mins
Total time: 20 mins

INGREDIENTS

- 2 medium eggs
- 1 small ripe banana
- 100 ml coconut milk
- 75 gr almond flour
- pinch of salt
- 1/2 tsp baking powder
- 1/4 tsp vanilla aroma
- 1/2 tsp cinnamon
- butter or oil for greasing
- optional: 1/2 tbsp psyllium fiber
- optional: Steviala sweetener to taste

PREPARATION METHOD

1. In a large bowl, combine the almond flour, salt, baking powder, vanilla taste, cinnamon, stevia sweetener, and psyllium fiber. Now take any other bowl and mash the banana with a fork. Add the coconut milk and eggs and beat till entire with a whisk.
2. Add the egg mixture to the flour aggregate and beat until smooth. Heat waffle iron and grease it with butter or oil. Add the batter and repeat till you have got made four waffles.

NUTRITIONAL VALUES

Serving Size: 1 wafer   Fat: 16.9   Proteins: 7.3
Calories: 208   Carbohydrates: 8.5

Cinnamon and coconut pancakes

Cooking time: 15 mins   **Total time: 20 mins**

INGREDIENTS

- 2 large eggs
- 1, 5 tablespoons coconut flour
- 1/2 tsp vanilla aroma
- 1/2 tsp cinnamon
- 3/4 tsp baking powder
- 1/2 banana mashed
- 60 ml coconut milk

PREPARATION METHOD

1. In a medium bowl, integrate the eggs, coconut milk, banana, and vanilla flavoring. Then take another bowl and mix inside the cinnamon, coconut flour, and baking powder. Then upload the flour mixture to the egg combination and mix it into a smooth batter.

2. Then take a small frying pan and heat a few butter or oil. Then take a tablespoon of batter and positioned it within the pan. As soon as bubbles shape on the floor of the pancake, turn it over (about a minute and a 1/2 baking). Bake for every other 30 seconds after turning and the pancake is prepared. Repeat this step until you run out of batter.

NUTRITIONAL VALUES

Serving Size: 1 pancake   Fats: 3.8   Proteins: 2.6
Calories: 58   Carbohydrates: 3.3

Chia pudding with coconut and strawberries

Cooking time: 10 mins   **Total time: 20 mins**

INGREDIENTS

- 250 ml unsweetened almond milk or coconut milk
- 3 tbsp chia seeds (25 g)
- 2 tbsp ground coconut
- 1 tsp vanilla aroma
- 1 handful of strawberries, cut into pieces
- Stevia or erythritol to taste

PREPARATION METHOD

1. In a large bowl, mix the almond milk, ground coconut, chia seeds, sweetener, and vanilla aroma properly with a whisk. Divide the mixture over 2 dishes and stand for 10 mins. Stir nicely from time to time throughout the ten minutes. Place the two bowls in the refrigerator in a single day or for at least 2 hours and location the strawberries on the pinnacle of the pudding earlier than serving.

NUTRITIONAL VALUES

Serving Size: 1 bowl   Fat: 18.5   Proteins: 9.4
Calories: 250   Carbohydrates: 3.8

Low-carbohydrate coconut porridge

Cooking time: 5 mins   **Total time: 10 mins**

INGREDIENTS

- 2 tbsp coconut flour
- optional: 2 tbsp linseed
- 180 ml of water or milk

- pinch of salt
- 1 large egg, beaten
- 2 tsp butter

- 1 tbsp coconut milk
- 1/2 tbsp Steviala Crystal

PREPARATION METHOD

Grab a small saucepan and add the coconut flour, flaxseed, salt, and water to it. Heat the contents of the pan over low heat, at the same time as stirring, until it starts evolved to thicken.

Then take the pan off the heat and upload half of the beaten egg. Stir properly, after which add the opposite half of. Then placed the pan again on the heat and warmth while stirring until it starts to take on the porridge structure. Then remove the pan from the warmth and add the butter, coconut milk, and Steviala Kristal whilst stirring. Pour the contents right into a bowl and serve with fresh fruit!

NUTRITIONAL VALUES

Serving Size: 1 small bowl   Fat: 19.5   Proteins: 11.6

Calories: 274   Carbohydrates: 5.5

Low-carbohydrate breakfast porridge

Cooking time: 10 mins   **Total time: 15 mins**

INGREDIENTS

- 140 ml almond milk, unsweetened
- 25 gr almond flour
- 2 tbsp coconut chips
- 1 tbsp flaxseed meal
- 1 tbsp chia seeds
- 1/2 tbsp erythritol or crystal sweet
- 1/2 tsp cinnamon
- 1/2 tsp vanilla aroma
- pinch of salt

PREPARATION METHOD

2. In a medium bowl, integrate the almond flour, coconut chips, flaxseed meal, chia seeds, erythritol, cinnamon, and salt.
3. Then pour the almond milk and vanilla aroma into a saucepan and add the bowl's dry substances. Bring the contents of the pan to a boil over high warmth.
4. When the porridge is boiling, reduce the warmth and simmer for 1 minute. Please make certain you do not overcook it because then the porridge will be too thick. After boiling, eliminate the pan from the warmth and permit it cool for three minutes.
5. Put the porridge in a bowl and garnish it with nuts, fruit, and coconut grater if favored. Enjoy your meal!

NUTRITIONAL VALUES

Serving Size: 1 bowl
Calories: 386

Fat: 32.5
Carbohydrates: 4.8

Fiber: 12.4
Proteins: 11.1

Low-carbohydrate cheese crackers

Cooking time: 10 mins
Total time: 25 mins

INGREDIENTS

- 170 gr grated mozzarella
- 85 gr almond flour
- 30 gr cream cheese
- 1 egg (M or L)
- 1/2 tsp sea salt
- 1/2 tsp dried rosemary or to taste

PREPARATION METHOD

1. Preheat the convection oven to 220 degrees. Then positioned the mozzarella, cream cheese, and almond flour in a massive microwave secure bowl.
2. Microwave the bowl for approximately 1 minute, until the cheese is in part melted. Then stir the contents of the bowl well with a spatula or fork.
3. Let the cheese and almond flour combination cool for 1-2 minutes. After cooling, upload the herbs and egg to the bowl and knead them together with your hands thru the dough for at least 1 minute.
4. Then positioned the dough between baking paper sheets and rolled the dough with a rolling pin to the preferred thickness. Remove the pinnacle sheet of baking paper and reduce the crackers into small squares (30 portions) with a pizza knife. You also can make big crackers if you desire.
5. Bake the cheese crackers in the preheated oven for 10-12 minutes. Keep a near eye on the oven; thin crackers will prepare dinner faster. After baking, permit the cheese crackers to cool for at least five mins on a cooling rack. You can preserve the crackers in a fresh container for 2-three days.

NUTRITIONAL VALUES

Serving Size: 1 mini cracker
Calories: 39

Fats: 3.1
Carbohydrates: 0.3

Proteins: 2.3

Low-carbohydrate crispbread

Cooking time: 5 mins   **Total time: 65 mins**

INGREDIENTS

- 100 gr sesame seeds
- 75 gr linseed
- 75 gr pine nuts
- 7 g of psyllium fiber
- 20 gr grated parmesan cheese
- 30 gr grated cheese
- 2 eggs
- 125 ml of water
- sea salt to taste

PREPARATION METHOD

1. Preheat the convection oven to 175 degree. Then integrate all components in a massive bowl and let the dough rest for five mins. Then take a baking tray and cowl it with a parchment paper
2. en. Then bake the crispbread inside the preheated oven for 20 minutes.
3. Lower the oven temperature to a hundred and forty degree and put off the baking tray from the oven. Cut the crispbread into 12 equally sized crackers and bake for another 35-forty mins at a hundred and forty degree.
4. After baking, open the oven door and allow the crispbread to cool inside the oven for at least 30 minutes. Serve the crackers with candy or savory toppings. Enjoy your meal!

NUTRITIONAL VALUES

Serving Size: 1 cracker   Fats: 12.1   Fiber: 3.0
Calories: 148   Carbohydrates: 1.2   Proteins: 7.4

Low-carbohydrate granola

Cooking time: 10 mins   **Total time: 30 mins**

INGREDIENTS

- 200 gr raw nut mix
- 80 gr coconut chips
- 40 gr pumpkin seeds
- 50 g linseed
- 50 gr sunflower seeds
- 1/2 tbsp cinnamon
- 50 gr coconut oil
- 1 tsp vanilla aroma
- 3 tbsp water
- optional: 3 tbsp sugar-free syrup

PREPARATION METHOD

1. Preheat the convection oven to one hundred sixty-five degrees. Melt the coconut oil in a saucepan. When the oil has melted, add the vanilla aroma, sugar-unfastened syrup, and water while stirring. Then do away with the pan from the warmth and set it aside.

2. In a massive bowl, combine the nuts, seeds, kernels, and cinnamon. Pour the oil aggregate over the nuts and stir properly into the granola. Divide the granola over a baking tray covered with parchment paper and bake the granola for 20-25 mins within the preheated oven. Toss the granola every five mins so that it does not burn.

3. After baking for 15 mins, add the coconut chips and fry for five-10 minutes. Let the granola calm down after baking and keep it in a big weck jar. Serve the granola with a part of complete-fats Greek yogurt. Enjoy your meal!

NUTRITIONAL VALUES

Serving Size: 1 portion (30 gr)   Fats: 18.6   Fiber: 2.0
Calories: 194   Carbohydrates: 1.9 Proteins: 4.7

Healthy fritt

Cooking time: 10 mins
Total time: 30 mins

INGREDIENTS

- 8 eggs
- 125 ml cream
- 125 gr grated cheese
- 250 gr mushrooms
- 100 g baby spinach
- 4 thick slices of bacon, fried
- 1 onion
- 2 cloves of garlic
- salt and pepper to taste
- paprika to taste
- chives to taste

PREPARATION METHOD

1. Preheat the convection oven to 190 degree and grease an oven dish (22x 22 cm) with a touch of olive oil. Then beat the eggs in a big bowl with the cooking cream, salt, paprika, and pepper. Add the grated cheese and mix well again.
2. On a huge reducing board, cut the onion into pieces, the mushrooms into slices, and crush the garlic. Then warmth a tablespoon of olive oil in a big frying pan and upload the chopped onion and beaten garlic. Fry for 1 minute and then add the mushrooms and fry for every other minute. Finally, add the spinach grade by grade and fry it inside three-four minutes.
3. Drain the extra liquid from the pan and add the contents to the greased oven dish. Divide it well over the dish after which pour the egg aggregate into the oven dish. Divide the bacon slices over the dish and area in the oven.
4. Bake the oven dish for 20-25 minutes in the preheated oven. Cut the oven dish into 4 pieces after baking and serve with arugula and chopped chives if desired. Enjoy your meal!

NUTRITIONAL VALUES

Serving Size: 1/4 of the dish
Calories: 330

Fats: 23.6
Carbohydrates: 3.8

Proteins: 24.7

Sugar free raspberry chia jam

Cooking time: 5 mins
Total time: 15 mins

INGREDIENTS

- 200 gr (frozen) raspberries
- 2 tbsp chia seeds
- 15 g erythritol

PREPARATION method

1. Add the clean or frozen raspberries to a saucepan alongside the erythritol. Place the saucepan on the fire and allow the raspberries to simmer for about five-10 mins over low heat at the same time as stirring. After simmering, stir well once more to break up all raspberries.
2. Prefer no seeds on your chia seeds? Then pour the mixture thru a colander and go back the juice to the saucepan. Then add the chia seeds whilst stirring and leave it at the hearth for about 1 minute, even as stirring.
3. Remove the pan from the heat and permit the jam to cool to room temperature. Then stir nicely again and then spoon the jam right into a preserving jar. The chia jam may be saved in the fridge for about 4 to five days. Enjoy your meal!

NUTRITIONAL VALUES

Serving Size: 15 gr (1/7)
Calories: 25
Fats: 1
Carbohydrates: 1.7
Proteins: 0.9

Low-carbohydrate chocolate cereal

Cooking time: 15 mins
Total time: 35 mins

INGREDIENTS

- 100 gr almond flour
- 50 gr walnuts
- 30 g linseed (brown or gold)
- 20 gr erythritol
- 10 gr cocoa powder
- 1 egg white
- 30 gr melted butter

PREPARATION METHOD

1. Preheat the convection oven to 175 degree. Add the almond flour, flaxseeds, walnuts, cocoa, and erythritol to a food processor or blender. Then grind it all first-class. After mixing, upload the melted butter and the egg white.
2. Mix well once more, and then flip off the system. Now use your arms to make small balls of the dough. Do you need to root them all equally? Then continually scoop a bit of dough with a small teaspoon.
3. Place a sheet of baking paper on a baking tray and area the balls. Bake the cereal balls inside the oven for 15 to twenty minutes. Then take the baking tray out of the oven and let the balls quiet down completely.
4. Store the low-carb breakfast cereal in a sealed field out of doors the refrigerator.

NUTRITIONAL VALUES

Serving size: 30 grams
Calories: 189

Fats: 17.1
Carbohydrates: 2.2

Fiber: 2.9
Proteins: 6.1

Chocolate chia pudding

Cooking time: 240 mins
Total time: 240 mins

INGREDIENTS

- Chia pudding
- 150 gr unsweetened almond milk
- 100 gr Greek yogurt
- 35 g chia seeds
- 1/2 tsp vanilla extract
- 10 gr cocoa
- 20 gr erythritol

Topping

- 15 gr finely chopped almonds
- 10 gr melted chocolate, milk or dark
- 1 tsp chia seeds

PREPARATION METHOD

1. In a huge bowl, blend the almond milk, Greek yogurt, chia seeds, cocoa powder, vanilla extract, and erythritol properly with a whisk.
2. Divide the pudding over 2 glasses and permit it to stand for 10 minutes. During the 10 minutes, you stir the entirety together well from time to time. Then positioned the two glasses inside the refrigerator for a minimum of four hours, ideally overnight.
3. If desired, you could garnish the pudding with topping. The chocolate is first-rate melted inside the au-bain-marie approach. You can hold the pudding inside the fridge for 2-3 days. With this recipe, you have got breakfast for 2 days!

NUTRITIONAL VALUES

Serving Size: 1 glass (1/2)   Fat: 16.6   Fiber: 8.5
Calories: 226   Carbohydrates: 4.3   Proteins: 9.6

Low-carb cinnamon crunchies

Cooking time: 20 mins
Total time: 45 mins

INGREDIENTS

- 100 gr almond flour
- 30 g linseed (blond or brown)
- 50 gr pecans
- 30 gr melted butter
- 1 egg white (from M egg)
- 30 g erythritol or to taste
- 2 tbsp cinnamon

PREPARATION METHOD

1. Preheat the convection oven to one hundred seventy-five degree. Add the almond flour, flaxseeds, pecans, cinnamon, and erythritol to your food processor. Then grind it all quality. Then upload the egg white and the melted butter. Then blend everything within the food processor into a dough.
2. Place the dough on a piece of parchment paper and then place a chunk of cling film or baking paper on top. Flatten the dough with your fingers and then roll it out with a rolling pin to a thickness of 0.5 cm. Remove the top layer of foil or baking paper and area the lowest sheet with the dough on a baking tray.
3. Bake the cinnamon crunchies for 18 mins in the preheated oven. Then take the baking tray out of the oven and reduce the baked dough lightly into small cubes. Then let it settle down absolutely. When the cinnamon crunchies have cooled completely, they are high-quality and crispy.
4. Keep the cinnamon cereal in a closed field in a non-humid location. You can hold them for at least per week to two weeks.

NUTRITIONAL VALUES

Serving Size: 30 gr crunchies   Fat: 15.4   Fiber: 2.6
Calories: 167   Carbohydrates: 1.1   Proteins: 4.6

MAIN COURSE
Low-carbohydrate bobotie

Cooking time: 40 mins
Total time: 40 mins

INGREDIENTS

- 250 gr green beans
- 125 gr mushrooms
- 300 gr ground beef, lean
- 1 small onion
- 1 clove of garlic
- 2 eggs
- 100 ml of whole milk
- 2 to 3 tsp curry
- 1 tsp cilantro
- 1/2 tsp ginger
- pinch of cinnamon
- 400 gr of cauliflower rice
- salt and pepper to taste

PREPARATION METHOD

1. Preheat the convection oven to 190 degree. Clean the green beans and remove the ends. Place a pan with water on it and pre-boil the green beans for about 5 mins. Meanwhile reduce the mushrooms, onion and garlic into small pieces.
2. Heat a tablespoon of olive oil in a frying pan and upload the chopped onion, garlic and curry, coriander, ginger, cinnamon, salt and pepper to the pan. Fry this in short and upload the minced meat after 2 mins. Fry the minced meat.
3. Then add the green beans and mushrooms and fry for a couple of minutes. Meanwhile beat the eggs with the milk. Spoon the contents of the pan into a small baking dish and pour the egg mixture over it.
4. Bake the bobotie for approx. 25 to 30 minutes inside the preheated oven. Just before the bobotie is prepared, fry the cauliflower rice in a wok till achieved and season with salt and pepper. Divide the rice and the dish between two plates and enjoy!

NUTRITIONAL VALUES

Serving Size: 1 portion (1/2 of the total)
Calories: 525
Fats: 29.9
Carbohydrates: 13.7
Proteins: 45.2

Leek curry casserole with minced meat

Cooking time: 15 mins
Total time: 35 mins

INGREDIENTS

- 500 gr of lean ground beef
- 125 gr bacon strips
- 4 stalks of leek
- 250 gr mushrooms
- 4 tsp curry powder
- 3 eggs (M)
- 100 ml of whipped cream
- 75 gr grated cheese
- salt and pepper to taste

PREPARATION METHOD

1. Preheat the convection oven to 190 degree.
2. Then add the smoked bacon strips to a frying pan and fry it till crispy. Drain the extra fat after which upload the ground red meat. Fry the minced meat.
3. In the period in-between, cut the mushrooms and leek into small portions and upload this to the frying pan at the side of the curry. Fry the veggies al dente while stirring constantly. Meanwhile beat the eggs in a big bowl with the whipped cream. Add the grated cheese and season with salt and pepper.
4. Put the leek-minced mixture in an oven dish and pour the crushed eggs over it. Bake the oven dish for approx. 25 mins within the preheated oven. Cut the dish into 4 pieces after baking and experience!

NUTRITIONAL VALUES

Serving Size: 1/4 of the dish
Calories: 595
Fats: 42.3
Carbohydrates: 8.7
Proteins: 42.8

Cauliflower quiche with cheese

Cooking time: 50 mins
Total time: 60 mins

INGREDIENTS

- 1 cauliflower
- 1/2 red onion
- 1 red pepper
- 125 gr bacon strips
- 100 gr grated cheese, matured
- 5 eggs (M)
- 125 gr crème fraîche
- paprika to taste
- salt and pepper to taste

1.

PREPARATION METHOD

2. Cut the cauliflower into small florets and add the florets to a pan full of water. Bring this to the boil and prepare dinner for the cauliflower florets for 10 minutes. In the intervening time, fry the bacon until crispy and permit the extra fat to drain after baking.
3. Chop the red onion and the bell pepper and fry it in short in a frying pan with olive oil. Now preheat the convection oven to a hundred ninety degree and grease a quiche pan nicely with butter. Then blend the eggs with the crème fraîche and grated cheese together nicely in a large bowl.
4. Now take the pan with the boiled cauliflower and let the water drain nicely. If necessary, pat the florets dry with a bit of kitchen paper. Add the cauliflower florets alongside the pre-fried bacon, bell pepper, and onion to the bowl with the eggs and stir till nicely blended.
5. Season the batter with salt, paprika, and pepper after which pour it into the greased quiche tin. Bake the cauliflower for approx. 35-40 minutes in the preheated oven until the filling has set. Then cut into 4 pieces and experience!

NUTRITIONAL VALUES

Serving Size: 1/4 of the quiche
Calories: 310
Fat: 24.4
Carbohydrates: 6.2
Proteins: 14.2

Low-carbohydrate goulash

Cooking time: 20 mins
Total time: 1800 mins

INGREDIENTS

- 700 gr of beef steak
- 1 onion
- 2 cloves of garlic
- 30 gr butter
- 1 red pepper
- 1 green pepper
- 400 gr canned tomatoes
- 1 tbsp tomato paste
- 400 gr pumpkin cubes, nutmeg
- 1 beef stock cube
- 200 ml of water
- 1 bay leaf
- 2 tsp paprika powder
- 1 tsp thyme
- 1 tsp caraway seeds
- pinch of black pepper
6.

PREPARATION METHOD

1. Cut the beef and onions into small portions and crush the garlic. Melt the butter in a casserole or skillet and upload the portions of meat. Brown the beef all around after which add the sliced onions and garlic. Bake this for a couple of minutes.
2. Meanwhile, cut the peppers into small pieces and upload this to the pan with the beef. Bake this for a few minutes too. Then upload the tomato paste and herbs to the pan whilst stirring. Deglaze with the water, stock dice, and tomato cubes.
3. Add the bay leaf to the pan and permit the goulash to simmer with the lid on for 2.5 hours over a low warmness. After 2.5 hours of simmering, add the pumpkin cubes and let it simmer for about half-hour, or till the pumpkin is cooked.
4. After simmering, divide the goulash into 4 portions and serve with cauliflower rice if desired. Enjoy your meal!

NUTRITIONAL VALUES

Serving Size: 1 bowl (1/4)
Calories: 401
Fat: 23.5
Carbohydrates: 8.7
Proteins: 34.8

Low-carbohydrate Shepherd's pie

Cooking time: 20 mins
Total time: 40 mins

INGREDIENTS

- Minced meat
- 1 small onion
- 2 cloves of garlic
- 1 carrot
- 1 tbsp olive oil
- 500 gr ground beef
- 1 zucchini
- 400 gr canned tomatoes
- 1 bay leaf
- 1/2 vegetable stock cube
- optional: 2 tsp arrowroot
- salt and pepper to taste

Topping

- 1 small cauliflower
- 20 butter, unsalted
- 50 ml whipped cream
- 50 gr grated cheese for oven gratin
- salt and pepper to taste

PREPARATION METHOD

1. Cut the onion and carrot into small portions and overwhelm the garlic. Heat a tablespoon of olive oil in a massive frying pan and upload the onion and garlic. Saute the onion and garlic until the onions begin to discolor. Then upload the sliced carrot and fry it for a few minutes.
2. Add the floor red meat to the pan and fry it while stirring. Meanwhile reduce the zucchini into small cubes. When the minced meat is cooked, add the zucchini, diced tomatoes, inventory cube, and bay leaf and let it simmer for 10 minutes over low heat, till the sauce has thickened. Then season the minced meat with salt and pepper. You can make the sauce thicker by including a 2 tsp arrowroot.
3. Now preheat the convection oven to one hundred seventy-five degree. Take the cauliflower and cut it into florets. Then bring a pan of water to a boil and add the cauliflower florets. Boil the florets for about 8-10 minutes.
4. Pour the contents of the pan into a colander and allow the florets to drain well. The drier the florets, the better the puree. Then return the drained florets to the pan. Then add the butter, whipped cream, cheese, salt, and pepper to the pan and blend this with a hand blender to an easy puree.
5. Remove the bay leaf from the pan with the minced meat and divide the minced meat over a big oven dish. Spoon the cauliflower puree over this and unfold the puree evenly over the dish with a spoon. Finally, sprinkle the dish with a little cheese
6. Bake the Shepherd pie for 25 minutes in the preheated oven. Cut the pie into 4 identical portions after baking and revel in!
7.

NUTRITIONAL VALUES

Serving size: 1/4 of the total
Calories: 452
Fats: 31.4

Carbohydrates: 10.8
Proteins: 29.4

Spicy chicken with cauliflower rice

Cooking time: 10 mins
Total time: 20 mins

INGREDIENTS

- 300 gr chicken cubes
- 1/2 onion
- 1 clove of garlic
- 3 tbsp sugar-free ketchup
- 2 tbsp soy sauce
- 1 to 2 tsp sambal oelek
- 2 tbsp peanut butter
- optional: 1 tbsp erythritol
- 2 tbsp water
- 400 gr of cauliflower rice
- 1 cucumber
- optional: fried onions

7.

PREPARATION METHOD

1. Cut the onion into small portions on a cutting board and weigh down the garlic. Add a tbsp olive oil to a frying pan and fry the onion and garlic in it. After approximately 2 minutes add the chook cubes and fry them all around.
2. When the chicken cubes are cooked and brown, upload the ketchup, soy sauce, sambal, peanut butter, and erythritol to the pan. Let the contents of the pan simmer for about five minutes, until the sauce has thickened. Add some water if the sauce becomes too thick
3. Meanwhile, fry the cauliflower rice in a separate pan. Cut the cucumber into slices and divide this over two plates together with the rice. Finally, divide the spicy bird over the plates and garnish with spring onions or fried onions. Enjoy your meal!
4.

NUTRITIONAL VALUES

Serving size: 1/2 of the total
Calories: 320
Fat: 8.5

Carbohydrates: 11.8
Proteins: 44.4

Low-carbohydrate hot dog sandwich

Cooking time: 10 mins
Total time: 40 mins

INGREDIENTS

Sandwiches

- 1 egg (M)
- protein from 1 egg (M)
- 100 gr almond flour
- 40 gr melted butter
- 2 tbsp psyllium fiber or 1 tbsp psyllium powder
- 1 tsp baking powder
- 1/2 tsp xanthan gum
- 1/4 tsp salt
- 60 ml of lukewarm water

hotdogs

- 3 fresh hot dogs or frankfurters
- 75 gr mixed raw vegetables with cabbage
- 1 tbsp olive oil
- mustard to taste
- sugar-free ketchup to taste

PREPARATION METHOD

1. Sandwiches. Preheat the convection oven to 175 degrees. Beat the whole egg and the whites together with an electric mixer. While blending, add the last ingredients for the sandwiches to the bowl. Beat the contents of the bowl into an easy or even dough.
2. Divide the dough into 3 balls and shape each ball right into a pistolet form with your fingers. If necessary, wet your fingers to make forming the bun-less complicated. Place the shaped balls on a baking tray coated with parchment paper and bake for 35 mins within the preheated oven.
3. Hotdog. After baking, let the buns calm down and then reduce a small notch inside the middle of the bun. Remove some of the dough inside the bun to make room for the hot canine. Prepare the hot dog or frankfurters in step with the commands on the package.
4. Divide the uncooked greens over the sandwiches and vicinity a warm canine in each sandwich. Garnish the hot canine with sugar-free ketchup, mustard, and every other sauce to taste. Serve and experience!

NUTRITIONAL VALUES

Serving Size: 1 hot dog sandwich
Calories: 547
Fat: 49.8

Carbohydrates: 4.0
Fiber: 6.1
Proteins: 19.7

Burrata salad with pesto

Cooking time: 10 mins
Total time: 20 mins

INGREDIENTS

- 150 gr burrata
- 100 gr arugula salad mix
- 150 gr cherry tomatoes
- 50 gr prosciutto

- 40 gr green pesto
- 1 tbsp olive oil
- handful of pine nuts
- 30 gr Parmesan cheese

8.

PREPARATION METHOD

1. Cut the Parma ham and cherry tomatoes into small pieces on a slicing board. Then, in a small bowl, blend the pesto and olive oil to make the dressing.
2. Divide the salad mixture over plates and beautify with the ham, cherry tomatoes, and parmesan cheese. Then cautiously reduce the burrata in half and vicinity it within the center of each plate.
3. Finally, in short toast the pine nuts in a frying pan and divide this over the plates along with the pesto dressing. Enjoy your meal!

9.

NUTRITIONAL VALUES

Serving size: 1/2 of the total
Calories: 490
Fats: 40.9

Carbohydrates: 7.1
Proteins: 21.8

Greek salad with chicken and tzaziki

Cooking time: 70 mins
Total time: 70 mins

INGREDIENTS

- Salad
- 300 gr chicken tenderloins
- 1/2 red onion
- 1 cucumber
- 3 tomatoes
- 12 olives
- 60 gr feta
- 100 gr tzatziki

- Chicken marinade
- 3 tbsp sour cream
- 1 clove of garlic, crushed
- 2 tbsp olive oil
- 1 tbsp lemon juice
- 2 tsp oregano
- 3/4 tsp salt
- 1/2 tsp black pepper

PREPARATION METHOD

1. In a huge bowl, combine the substances for the chicken marinade. Add the hen breast strips to the bowl and cover with hold film. Put the bowl in the refrigerator and permit the marinade to soak for a minimum of an hour.
2. Heat a tablespoon of olive oil in a frying pan or grease a grill with a bit of oil. Place the strips with a spatula inside the frying pan or grill and bake them for about 6-eight minutes.
3. Meanwhile, reduce the cucumber and tomato into cubes. Then take the red onion and cut it into cubes or earrings. Divide the vegetables among bowls and add the feta, olives, and tzatziki.
4. Let the chicken strips calm down after baking and then upload them to the bowl. Garnish the salad with a bit of sparkling parsley if desired. Enjoy your meal!

Mexican meatballs

Cooking time: 10 mins
Total time: 20 mins

INGREDIENTS

- Meatballs
- 500 gr ground beef
- 1 tbsp almond flour
- 1 jalapeño pepper
- 85 grams of grated cheddar
- 1 egg (M)
- 1 clove of garlic pressed
- 2 tsp cumin
- 2 tsp chili powder
- 1 tsp paprika powder
- 1/2 tsp salt
- Salsa
- 1 can of peeled tomatoes (400 gr)
- 1 jalapeño pepper, finely chopped
- 1/2 onion, finely chopped
- 1 clove of garlic, crushed

- lime juice to taste
- 1 tsp cumin
- 1 tsp salt
- handful of parsley, finely chopped

PREPARATION METHOD

1. Meatballs. Preheat the convection oven to one hundred ninety ranges. Cut the jalapeño pepper into small pieces on a large reducing board. Add the chopped pepper to a large bowl in conjunction with the remaining meatball elements.
2. Mix the substances nicely with your arms inside the bowl. Shape the minced meat into approx. 15 meatballs. Place the balls on a baking tray protected with parchment paper. Bake the balls for about 20 mins in the preheated oven.
3. Salsa. Meanwhile, make the salsa by way of including all of the salsa ingredients in a blender. Turn at the blender till the salsa has the preferred consistency. Add the salsa to a bowl and placed it blanketed within the refrigerator for some time.
4. Serve the meatballs with salsa and sour cream and spring onion if favored. Enjoy your meal!

NUTRITIONAL VALUES

Serving Size: 1 meatball with salsa
Calories: 95
Fat: 5.8

Carbohydrates: 1.5
Proteins: 8.9

Smoked chicken salad

Cooking time: 15 mins
Total time: 20 mins

INGREDIENTS

- Salad
- 100 gr salad mix
- 150 gr smoked chicken fillet slices
- 2 vine tomatoes
- 100 gr bacon strips
- 150 gr mini mozzarella balls

- 1/2 cucumber
- Yogurt mayonnaise dressing
- 4 tbsp whole yogurt
- 2 tbsp mayonnaise
- 1 tsp mustard

PREPARATION METHOD

1. Cut the tomatoes and cucumber into small cubes on a large slicing board. Then warmness a frying pan over medium warmth and upload the bacon. Fry the bacon for approximately 5 mins until golden brown and crispy.
2. Add the salad blend, smoked chicken, and mini mozzarella balls to a massive bowl. Mix the entirety together nicely and upload the chopped vegetables and the cooled bacon cubes.
3. Now make the dressing by using mixing the yogurt, mayonnaise, and mustard nicely in a bowl. Divide the salad between plates and serve with a yogurt mayonnaise dressing. Enjoy your meal!

NUTRITIONAL VALUES

Serving Size: 1 portion (1/2 of the total)
Calories: 506
Fat: 36.0

Carbohydrates: 5.4
Proteins: 39.5

Salmon teriyaki with broccoli rice

Cooking time: 15 mins
Total time: 25 mins

INGREDIENTS

Salmon teriyaki

- 2 salmon fillets
- 50 ml soy sauce
- 50 ml of water
- 1 clove of garlic, finely crushed
- 3 cm fresh ginger, grated
- 1 tbsp wok oil
- 1 tsp arrowroot
- optional: 1 tbsp erythritol
- 1 tbsp sesame seeds

10. Broccoli rice

- 400 gr broccoli rice
- 1 tbsp olive oil
- 1 shallot
- 2 lemon slices
- 1 stalk of spring onion
- salt and pepper to taste

PREPARATION METHOD

1. Preheat the oven to 180 degree. In a small saucepan, combine the soy sauce, beaten garlic, grated ginger, wok oil, arrowroot, and water. Put the pan at the range and convey it to a boil. Let it boil for approximately 2-three minutes until the sauce has thickened slightly.
2. Place the salmon fillets in a small oven dish and pour the sauce over the salmon fillets. Now take a spoon or kitchen brush and coat the zam fillets properly with the sauce in the dish. Bake the salmon teriyaki within the preheated oven for 15 minutes.
3. Meanwhile, finely chop a shallot and fry it in a frying pan with olive oil. Add the broccoli rice and wok it inside four-5 mins. Season the rice with salt and pepper. Divide the broccoli rice between plates and set aside.
4. After baking, location the salmon fillets on the broccoli rice and garnish with chopped spring onions and sesame seeds. Serve the salmon fillets with a slice of lemon if favored. Enjoy your meal!

NUTRITIONAL VALUES

Serving size: 1/2 of the total
Calories: 530
Proteins: 38.4

Fats: 37.8
Carbohydrates: 5.4

Fish dish with tomato sauce

Cooking time: 30 mins
Total time: 45 mins

INGREDIENTS

- 1 cauliflower
- 1 vegetable stock cube
- 2 tins of peeled tomatoes (800 gr)
- 2 cloves of garlic, finely crushed
- 4 tbsp olive oil
- 500 grams of cod
- 250 gr mozzarela (bulb)
- 1/2 lemon
- 1 sprig of parsley
- salt and pepper to taste

PREPARATION METHOD

1. Preheat the oven to two hundred degree. Add the peeled canned tomatoes to a big stockpot and mash it finely with a hand blender. Season the tomato sauce with salt and pepper and upload 2 tbsp olive oil and the beaten garlic. Bring the sauce to the boil and cook for about five-10 mins, until the sauce has thickened properly.
2. Meanwhile, reduce the cauliflower into florets and upload the florets to a pan full of water. Add the inventory dice and bring the water to a boil. Cook the cauliflower for approx. 10 minutes until al dente and then permit the water drain.
3. Add the tomato sauce to a big casserole dish and place the cod within the sauce. Season the cod and sauce with salt and pepper. Then additionally upload the cauliflower florets. Tear the mozzarella into small portions and spread calmly over the dish.
4. Bake the fish dish in the preheated oven for 25-30 minutes. Meanwhile, grate the lemon and finely chop the parsley. Add this together with the last olive oil to a bowl and blend properly. After baking, divide the dish into four portions and serve with the lemon olive oil.

NUTRITIONAL VALUES

Serving Size: 1/4 of the dish
Calories: 400
Fats: 23.6

Carbohydrates: 9.3
Proteins: 35.3

Chicken jambalaya with cauliflower rice

Cooking time: 15 mins
Total time: 30 mins

INGREDIENTS

- 300 gr chicken fillet
- 125 gr chorizo
- 1 onion
- 1 clove of garlic
- 1/2 red bell pepper
- 1 tbsp tomato paste
- 2 large tomatoes
- 1 tsp paprika powder
- 1 tsp cajun seasoning
- salt and pepper to taste
- parsley to taste
- 600 gr cauliflower rice

PREPARATION METHOD

1. Cut the onion into small pieces and weigh down the garlic. Then cut the bird breast and chorizo into small cubes and set them aside. Heat a tbsp olive oil in a large wok pan and fry the onion and garlic in it until the onion starts off evolved to discolor. Then add the chicken and herbs and fry the chicken till done.
2. In the intervening time, cut the bell pepper and tomato into small cubes and add this to the chicken together with the chorizo. Fry this in short and then add a tablespoon of tomato puree to the pan. Fry the contents of the pan inside approx. Five mins even as stirring.
3. Meanwhile, fry the cauliflower rice in every other pan. Add this to the pan with the hen and chorizo and fry it in short. Divide the bird jambalaya between 3 plates and season with salt, pepper, and sparkling parsley. Enjoy your meal!

NUTRITIONAL VALUES

Serving Size: 1 portion (1/3)
Calories: 347
Fat: 16.6Carbohydrates: 9.8
Fiber: 5.1
Proteins: 36.8

Chicken siam with cauliflower rice

Cooking time: 15 mins
Total time: 25 mins

INGREDIENTS

- 500 gr chicken fillet cubes
- 400 gr of cauliflower rice
- 1 red pepper
- 2 cloves of garlic
- 1 cm ginger
- 1/2 onion
- 3 tbsp olive oil
- 3 tbsp oyster sauce
- 1 tbsp soy sauce
- 50 ml of water
- 2 tsp arrowroot
- 2 stalks of spring onion
- 40 gr cashew nuts

PREPARATION METHOD

1. Finely chop the ginger and onion on a slicing board. Then warmness the olive oil in a massive frying pan. Add the chook cubes and stir-fry for about 3-6 minutes till accomplished. Then crush the garlic and upload it to the pan along with the onion and ginger. Fry the seasonings for three minutes.
2. In the interim, reduce the bell pepper into small pieces after which upload this to the pan. In a small bowl, mix the water, oyster sauce, and soy sauce together and add this to the chicken and vegetables.
3. Then mix in a tumbler a tbsp water with 2 tsp arrowroot and upload this to the pan to thicken the sauce. Boil the contents of the pan for 2-3 mins, until the sauce has thickened. Finally, stir the cashews into the pan.
4. Now warmth a tbsp olive oil in a new pan and wok the cauliflower rice till accomplished. Finely chop the spring onion and set it apart. Divide the cauliflower rice over four plates and spoon the hen siam over it. Garnish with the sliced spring onion. Enjoy your meal!

NUTRITIONAL VALUES

Serving size: 1/4 of the total
Calories: 308
Fats: 13.7
Carbohydrates: 9.8
Proteins: 34.2

Stuffed zucchini with pizza topping

Cooking time: 15 mins
Total time: 25 mins

INGREDIENTS

- 2 courgettes
- 200 gr tomato sauce
- 1/4 red onion
- 1/2 green pepper
- 125 gr mushrooms
- 60 gr salami
- 80 gr grated mozzarella
- Italian herbs to taste
- salt and pepper to taste

PREPARATION METHOD

1. Preheat the convection oven to two hundred degrees. Wash the courgettes and cut them in half lengthwise. Remove the flesh with a spoon and set it aside. Then cut the green pepper, mushrooms, onion, and salami into small pieces.
2. Take the zucchini and place it in a greased oven dish. Fill the 4 hollowed-out courgettes with the tomato sauce. Then divide the sliced veggies and salami over the courgettes. Season the crammed zucchini with Italian herbs, salt, and pepper.
3. Finally, sprinkle the courgettes with grated mozzarella and cowl the dish with aluminum foil. Bake the courgettes in the preheated oven for 15 mins. Then remove the foil and bake for every other 10 minutes.

NUTRITIONAL VALUES

Serving Size: 2 pieces of stuffed zucchini
Calories: 338
Fats: 19.6
Carbohydrates: 15.8
Proteins: 22.3

Lettuce wraps with Mexican chicken

Cooking time: 10 mins
Total time: 70 mins

INGREDIENTS

Chicken marinade

- 300 gr chicken fillet
- 2 tbsp olive oil
- 1 tbsp lime juice
- 1 tbsp Taco seasoning
- 1/2 tsp ground coriander
- 1/2 tsp dried oregano
- salt and pepper to taste
- wraps
- 1 head of romaine lettuce
- 1 avocado
- 1/2 red onion
- 1/2 cucumber
- 250 gr cherry tomatoes

Sauce

- 125 ml of sour cream
- 1 tbsp mayonnaise
- handful of fresh parsley
- 1/2 tbsp lime juice
- 1/4 tsp cumin powder
- 1/4 tsp garlic powder

PREPARATION METHOD

1. In a huge bowl, mix the herbs properly collectively for the marinade. Add the olive oil and blend properly once more. Cut the chicken into cubes if essential and add this to the marinade. Put the bowl inside the fridge and allow the marinade to soak for at least an hour.
2. Meanwhile, in a bowl, mix all the substances for the sauce collectively with a whisk. Cover the bowl with cling movie and placed it in the fridge. Then reduce the avocado, cucumber, cherry tomatoes, and onion into small portions.
3. Then take the bowl with the chicken from the refrigerator. Heat a tablespoon of olive oil in a frying pan and add the bird and marinade to the pan. Fry the hen in approximately 10 mins until brown and done.
4. Place some of the lettuce leaves in a row on a huge shelf and fill them with the sliced greens and chicken. Garnish with the sauce and serve. Enjoy your meal!

NUTRITIONAL VALUES

Serving Size: 2 lettuce wraps
Calories: 359
Fats: 22.8

Carbohydrates: 7.4
Proteins: 28.4

Avocado salad with chicken

Cooking time: 30 mins
Total time: 30 mins

INGREDIENTS

Chicken

- 300 gr chicken fillet (cubes)
- 1 tbsp olive oil
- 1/2 tsp salt and black pepper
- 1/4 tsp paprika powder
- 1/8 tsp onion powder
- 1/4 tsp garlic powder
- 1/8 tsp cumin powder
- 1/4 tsp chili powder
- 1/8 tsp oregano
- lemon juice from 1/2 lemon

Salad

- 1 cucumber
- 1 avocado
- 250 gr cherry tomatoes
- 1/4 red onion
- 3 tbsp lime juice
- 2 tbsp olive oil
- salt and pepper to taste

PREPARATION METHOD

1. In a large bowl, blend all the herbs for the marinade collectively with olive oil and lemon juice. Add the chook fillet (cubes) to the bowl and put it inside the refrigerator. Let the marinade sit down for at least 15 mins.
2. Fry the marinated hen in a frying pan, grill pan, or at the barbecue. In the intervening time, reduce the cucumber, avocado, and cherry tomatoes into pieces. Chop the onion and upload the vegetables to a bowl.
3. After baking, reduce the chicken fillet into cubes and upload it to the bowl with the vegetables. Mix the contents of the bowl nicely. Then make the dressing by mixing the lime juice and olive oil in a small bowl.
4. Divide the salad among two plates and serve with the fresh lime dressing. Enjoy your meal!

NUTRITIONAL VALUES

Serving size: 1/2 of the total

Calories: 438

Fat: 13.0

Carbohydrates: 8.4

Fiber: 5.7

Proteins: 39.1

Indian curry casserole

Cooking time: 40 mins
Total time: 60 mins

INGREDIENTS

Casserole

- 600 gr chicken thigh fillet
- 1 cauliflower
- 2 tbsp olive oil
- 1 tin of diced tomatoes (400 gr)
- 200 ml coconut milk
- 1 tbsp tomato paste
- 1/2 cube of chicken stock
- salt and pepper to taste
- 100 g baby spinach
- 200 gr green beans

Curry paste

- 2 tbsp grated ginger
- 1/2 onion
- 2 cloves of garlic
- 1 tsp ground cumin
- 1 tsp turmeric
- coriander to taste
- 1/2 tsp paprika
- 1/2 tsp garam masala
- 1 red pepper, finely chopped

PREPARATION METHOD

1. Preheat the convection oven to one hundred eighty degrees. Cut the cauliflower into florets. Bring a pan of water to the boil and cook the cauliflower for 5 mins until soft. After cooking, let it drain properly and location it in a greased oven dish together with the bird thigh fillet. Drizzle the cauliflower and chook with olive oil and season with salt and pepper. Bake the dish for approx. 25 minutes in the preheated oven.

2. Meanwhile, make the curry paste by mixing all of the elements in a blender. Add the curry paste to a skillet and cook dinner for 1 minute. Then upload a tbsp olive oil and fry for every other minute. Then take the tomato paste, diced tomatoes, coconut milk, and the chicken stock and add this to the curry paste. Let this simmer for 5 mins over low heat whilst stirring. Taste the sauce and add more salt or pepper if important.

3. Stir fry the spinach in a frying pan for two-three minutes and upload it to the sauce. Remove the casserole with the fried chicken from the oven and take a look at if the chicken is cooked. Add the curry sauce and bake the dish for another 10 minutes within the preheated oven.

4. Meanwhile, carry a pan of water to a boil and add the green beans. Cook the green beans for 5-10 mins al dente. Serve the curry dish with the cooked green beans and a bit of Greek yogurt if favored. Enjoy your meal!

NUTRITIONAL VALUES

Serving Size: 1/4 of the dish

Calories: 402

Fats: 23.9

Carbohydrates: 9.3

Fiber: 6.4

Proteins: 34.4

Teriyaki chicken with cauliflower rice

Cooking time: 20 mins
Total time: 40 mins

INGREDIENTS

Marinade

- 1 tbsp wok oil
- 1 clove of garlic,
- 3 cm fresh ginger
- 1 tbsp sesame seeds
- 30 ml soy sauce
- 30 ml of water
- 1 tbsp erythritol
- optional 1/4 tsp xanthan gum

Teriyaki

- 300 gr chicken fillet cubes
- 400 gr broccoli florets
- 1 tbsp wok oil
- 1/2 onion
- 250 gr sliced mushrooms

- 400 gr of cauliflower rice
- 1 stalk of spring onion
- 2 tbsp sesame seeds
- optional: 1 red pepper

PREPARATION METHOD

1. Using a garlic press, press the clove of garlic into a pulp. Then take a small grater and grate the ginger with it. Heat a tablespoon of wok oil in a massive frying pan and upload the garlic, ginger, and sesame seeds. Fry this for 1 minute over an excessive warmness and then upload the soy sauce, water, and erythritol. Reduce warmth and simmer for 2 mins. Finally, upload the xanthan gum and heat it until the sauce has thickened.

2. Let the marinade settle down and then upload it to a bowl in conjunction with all of the chicken cubes. Cover the bowl and let the marinade relax in the fridge for at least 15 mins.

3. Meanwhile, finely chop the onion and heat a tablespoon of wok oil in a big frying pan. Add the onion to the pan and fry it till it starts to discolor. Spoon the hen with the marinade into the pan and fry all of it round until carried out and golden brown.

4. Add the sliced mushrooms and fry for 2-three mins. Add a finely chopped pink pepper for greater highly spiced teriyaki. In the period in-between, carry a pan of water to the boil and add the broccoli florets. Boil the florets with a lid on the pan for 3-4 minutes till gentle.

5. Then take every other frying pan and wok the cauliflower rice until accomplished. Divide the chicken teriyaki, cauliflower rice, and cooked broccoli among plates and garnish with chopped spring onion and sesame seeds. Enjoy your meal!

NUTRITIONAL VALUES

Serving size: 1/2 of the total
Calories: 431
Fats: 16.2

Carbohydrates: 9.4
Fiber: 12.2
Proteins: 51.5

Low-carbohydrate enchiladas

Cooking time: 25 mins

Total time: 50 mins

INGREDIENTS

Cauliflower tortillas

- 400 gr of cauliflower rice
- 3 eggs (M)
- 1/2 tsp salt
- 1/4 tsp black pepper

Enchilada sauce

- 3 tbsp olive oil
- 2 tbsp arrowroot powder
- 1 can of tomato pulp or cubes
- 350 ml of water
- 1/2 vegetable stock cube
- 1/2 tsp chili powder
- 1/4 tsp ground cumin
- 1/4 tsp garlic powder
- salt and pepper to taste

Stuffing

- 500 gr chicken fillet
- 150 gr mozzarella

PREPARATION METHOD

1. For approximately 20 minutes. Remove the bird breasts from the pan and pull them aside with spoons to make pulled chook.
2. Preheat the convection oven to a hundred and eighty degree. Heat a tablespoon of olive oil in a large frying pan and upload the cauliflower rice. Wok the rice for about 3 minutes. Add the rice to an easy tea towel or cheesecloth and let it quiet down. Then squeeze the moisture out of the rice and add the rice to a bowl.
3. Add the eggs, salt, and pepper to the bowl and mix nicely. Cover a baking tray with parchment paper and scoop eight piles onto the baking tray. Form 8 tortillas from the mounds and bake for 10 minutes inside the preheated oven. Then flip the tortillas and bake for every other 5 minutes. If all the tortillas do not suit the plate, you can bake it in. Then fry the tortillas in the frying pan for two minutes for a brown crust.
4. Heat three tbsp olive oil in a pan and upload the arrowroot and chili powder. Fry this for two mins even as stirring after which upload the tomato pulp, water, and other herbs. Reduce warmth and simmer for 10 minutes.
5. Take the casserole and grease it with oil. Add a few tablespoons of sauce and region tortillas on top. Then upload the pulled bird, cheese, and a touch sauce. Repeat this till all components are used.
6. Cover the dish with aluminum foil and bake for 30 minutes in the preheated oven. Remove the foil from the dish and bake for any other five mins. Divide the enchiladas among four plates and serve with spring onion, crème fraîche, and guacamole if desired.

NUTRITIONAL VALUES

Serving Size: 1/4 of the dish

Calories: 420

Fat: 45.9

Carbohydrates: 10.1

Proteins: 45.9

Stuffed portobello with goat cheese

Cooking time: 30 mins
Total time: 40 mins

INGREDIENTS

- 4 portobellos
- 2 shallots
- 2 cloves of garlic
- dash of olive oil
- 100 g baby spinach
- 200 gr tomato pulp or cubes
- 1 tbsp Italian herbs
- 100 gr goat cheese
- handful of chopped walnuts
- salt and pepper to taste
- optional: spring onion

PREPARATION
METHOD

1. Heat the convection oven to two hundred degree. Cover a baking tray with parchment paper and lightly grease it with a touch of olive oil. Clean the portobello mushrooms with a paper towel and carefully cast off the stem. Then vicinity the mushrooms with the stem dealing with up at the baking tray. Spread the mushrooms with olive oil and season with salt and pepper to taste. Bake the portobello mushrooms inside the preheated oven for 10-15 minutes.

2. In the period in-between, reduce the shallots into small pieces and weigh down the garlic with a garlic press. Heat a tablespoon of olive oil in a big frying pan and add half of the sliced shallot and crushed garlic. Fry for a minute, till the onion starts to discolor. Then add the spinach and fry for 2-three minutes. Season with salt and pepper and set aside.

3. Now take a brand-new pan and fry the relaxation of the chopped shallot and crushed garlic in it. Add the tomato pulp or diced tomatoes and cook for 5-10 minutes, till the sauce has decreased and thickened. Season the sauce with salt, pepper, and Italian herbs.

4. Remove the portobello mushrooms from the oven and pat them dry with a paper towel. Then divide the tomato sauce evenly over the mushrooms. Add the spinach and eventually the chunks of goat cheese. Bake the portobello mushrooms within the preheated oven for every other 15 mins.

5. After baking for 10 mins, upload chopped walnuts and cook dinner for any other five mins. After baking, garnish the stuffed portobello mushrooms with finely chopped spring onion. Enjoy your meal!

NUTRITIONAL VALUES

Serving Size: 2 stuffed portobello mushrooms
Calories: 345
Fats: 24.1

Carbohydrates: 13.4
Proteins: 16.2

Pad thai with zucchini noodles

Cooking time: 10 mins
Total time: 20 mins

INGREDIENTS

- 2 courgettes or 400 gr courgetti
- 2 tbsp olive oil
- 3 shallots
- 1 clove of garlic
- 3 eggs
- 1 - 2 tbsp soy sauce
- juice of 1 lime
- 1 tbsp tamarind paste
- 1 tsp fish sauce or Worcestershire sauce
- dried red pepper flakes to taste
- 125 gr bean sprouts
- 4 tbsp peanuts
- optional: fresh cilantro

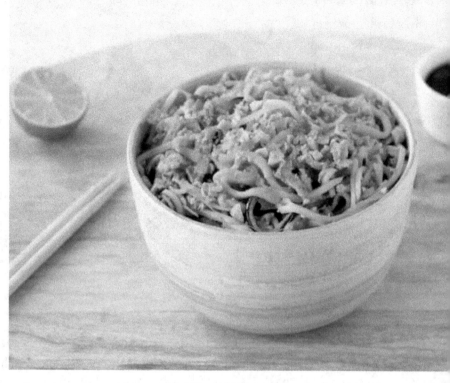

PREPARATION METHOD

1. In a small bowl, integrate the soy sauce, lime juice, fish sauce, tamarind, and red pepper flakes. Set apart. Clean the courgettes and remove the ends. Use a spiral cutter to make noodles from the zucchini or use prepared-made zucchini spaghetti
2. Then warmness a tablespoon of olive oil in a big wok pan and upload the zucchini spaghetti to the pan. Fry the zucchini spaghetti over excessive warmth for about 2-3 minutes. In the period in-between, reduce the shallots into small pieces and weigh down the garlic.
3. Let the zucchini spaghetti cool for 5 mins after which pour the contents of the pan into a colander. Let the excess moisture drain properly. Then easy the wok pan and upload a tablespoon of olive oil to the pan. Return to the heat and upload the sliced shallots and crushed garlic. Fry for two mins, until the onion begins to discolor.
4. Meanwhile, beat the eggs in a bowl and add this to the pan. Let the egg set a bit and then stir well with a spatula via the pan to make a stirring egg. Add the homemade sauce, bean sprouts, and zucchini spaghetti to the eggs and fry for 2 mins.
5. Divide the contents of the pan among 3 bowls and garnish with the chopped peanuts and fresh coriander.

NUTRITIONAL VALUES

Serving size: 1/3 of the total
Calories: 270
Fat: 17.5

Carbohydrates: 12.3
Fiber: 4.1
Proteins: 13.8

Oven dish with spinach and minced meat

Cooking time: 20 mins
Total time: 40 mins

INGREDIENTS

Casserole:

- 300 gr of lean ground beef
- 3 slave finches
- 1 onion
- 1 red pepper
- 250 gr mushrooms
- 1 clove of garlic
- 400 gr of cauliflower rice
- 350 gr frozen spinach
- 2 tomatoes
- 50 grated cheese for oven gratin
- salt and pepper to taste
- optional: chili powder and garlic powder

Cheese sauce:

- 200 ml of cooking cream
- 50 gr cream cheese
- 2 tbsp butter
- 50 gr grated cheddar cheese
- 1/2 tsp mustard
- salt and pepper to taste

PREPARATION METHOD.

1. Preheat the oven to 180 degrees. Then reduce the mushrooms, onion, and bell pepper into small portions. Heat a bit of oil in a frying pan and upload the sliced onion. Press the garlic the usage of a garlic press and upload this to the pan. Fry this for 1-2 mins, until the onion starts off evolved to discolor.

2. Add the minced meat and fry it lose. Season the minced meat with salt, pepper, and other spices to flavor. Finally, upload the sliced bell pepper and mushrooms and fry for three mins. After baking, drain the extra liquid and set the pan apart.

3. Heat the frozen spinach in a saucepan over low heat until it's miles warm. Then take every other frying pan and add a tablespoon of butter. Heat the butter and location the salad finches within the pan. Fry the slave finches over low heat for approximately 20 minutes.

4. Then take another frying pan and wok the cauliflower rice in it for two-three minutes. Season the rice with a touch of salt and pepper. Now take the pan with the spinach and permit the excess moisture to drain. Add the spinach to the pan with the cauliflower rice and stir properly.

5. Then upload the cauliflower and spinach combination to the minced meat and stir properly. Cut the tomatoes into slices and eliminate the salad finches from the pan while they're cooked. Cut the slave finches into slices.

6. Now make the cheese sauce in a saucepan. To do this, add the cooking cream, cream cheese, and butter to the pan. Heat this over low heat, while stirring, until the whole lot has melted. Add the grated cheddar and season with mustard, salt, and pepper. Stir nicely and set aside.

7. Now take the oven dish and scoop 1/2 of the minced meat aggregate on the bottom. Divide half of the tomato and salad finch slices over it. Pour a touch of cheese sauce on pinnacle and sprinkle with grated cheese.

8. Repeat the above step until you run out of substances. Bake the casserole for 15-20 minutes inside the preheated oven, until the cheese is golden brown. After baking, divide the dish into four portions. Enjoy your meal!

NUTRITIONAL VALUES

Serving Size: 1/4 of the dish

Calories: 682

Fat: 49.8

Carbohydrates: 11.6

Fiber: 6.3

Proteins: 43.7

Low-carb cauliflower lasagna

Cooking time: 20 mins
Total time: 70 mins

INGREDIENTS

Cauliflower lasagne sheets:

- 400 gr of cauliflower rice
- 15 gr Parmesan cheese
- 2 eggs
- salt and pepper to taste

Bolognese sauce:

- 500 gr (lean) ground beef
- 1 onion
- 1 clove of garlic
- 250 gr mushrooms

- 400 gr diced tomatoes or pulp
- 1 tbsp Italian herbs
- 1 tbsp tomato paste
- salt and pepper to taste
- Ricotta Sauce and Lasagna:
- 250 gr ricotta
- 1 egg
- 25 gr grated Parmesan cheese
- 65 gr grated mozzarella
- salt and pepper to taste

PREPARATION METHOD

Lasagne sheets:

1. Preheat the oven to one hundred ninety degree. Cover a baking tray with parchment paper and grease it with a bit of olive oil. Then warmth a bit of oil in a frying pan and upload the cauliflower rice. Season with salt and pepper and stir-fry the rice within four mins.
2. Place the cauliflower rice in a smooth kitchen towel and squeeze out all the moisture. Then upload the cauliflower rice to a bowl with the eggs, parmesan cheese, salt, and pepper. Mix properly and divide the combination over the baking tray with parchment paper.
3. Bake the cauliflower lasagne sheets for 15 mins within the preheated oven and permit them to cool for 10 minutes after baking. Cut into 6 even-sized sheets and set them apart.

Bolognese Sauce And Lasagna:

1. Preheat the oven to a hundred and sixty ranges. Cut the onion and mushrooms into small pieces and overwhelm the garlic. Heat a touch little bit of olive oil in a large frying pan and upload the chopped onion and crushed garlic. Bake for 1 minute until the onion starts off evolved to discolor. Then placed the mushrooms in the pan and fry for 2 minutes.
2. Add the ground beef and fry it till finished. Finally add the tomato pulp, puree, Italian herbs, salt, and pepper. Let the sauce simmer for 10-15 minutes without a lid.
3. Meanwhile, in a bowl, combine the ricotta, egg, and a handful of parmesan cheese. Then take an oven dish and grease it with oil.
4. Spoon a few serving spoons of bolognese sauce into the dish. Place some cauliflower lasagne sheets on top and spread this ricotta sauce. Sprinkle this with a touch of parmesan cheese and mozzarella. Repeat this till all components are used.
5. Cover the dish with aluminum foil and bake for 25 minutes in the preheated oven. Then take away the foil and bake for another 15 mins. Cut the lasagna into 4 portions and experience!

NUTRITIONAL VALUES

Serving Size: 1/4 of the lasagna

Calories: 528

Fat: 32.4

Carbohydrates: 11.4

Fiber: 4.2

Proteins: 46.4

Swedish meatballs

Cooking time: 15 mins
TOTAL TIME: 25 MINS

INGREDIENTS

Meatballs:

- 300 gr of lean ground beef
- 1 small egg
- 2 tbsp finely chopped onion
- 25 ml whipped cream
- 1 tbsp coconut flour
- 1 tbsp dried parsley
- 1/2 tsp garlic powder
- pinch of nutmeg
- salt and pepper to taste
- 2 tbsp butter

Cream sauce:

- 150 ml unsalted beef stock
- 75 ml whipped cream
- 35 gr cream cheese

- 1/2 tsp Worcestershire sauce
- 1/2 tbsp mustard
- salt and pepper to taste

PREPARATION METHOD

1. In a large bowl, blend the minced meat with the finely chopped onion, whipped cream, coconut flour, herbs, and egg collectively with a spatula. Then mix nicely together with your hands once more and form 15 small meatballs from the minced meat.
2. Melt the butter in a massive skillet and lightly upload the meatballs. Fry the meatballs over a low warmness for about 10 minutes. Stir them sometimes all through baking in order that they cook dinner frivolously.
3. Remove the meatballs from the pan and quickly place them on a plate. Heat the cream cheese within the microwave or in a small pan for 1 minute. Add 1/2 of the beef stock to the pan with the meatball gravy and warm it over medium warmth. Add the melted cream cheese and the whipped cream whilst stirring and cook for a minute.
4. Pour the sauce from the pan into a blender and add the relaxation of the beef stock. Run the blender in brief, until the sauce is well blended. Return the sauce to the pan and add the mustard and Worcestershire sauce. Simmer the sauce over low heat for 5-10 mins till thickened to your liking.
5. Heat the meatballs briefly in a separate pan and divide among two plates. Serve the meatballs with the cream sauce and garnish with parsley. Enjoy your meal!

NUTRITIONAL VALUES

Serving Size: 5 meatballs
Calories: 388
Fat: 32.0

Carbohydrates: 2.7
Proteins: 22.8

Big Mac casserole

Cooking time: 10 mins
Total time: 30 mins

INGREDIENTS

Casserole:

- 500 gr of lean ground beef
- 1 onion
- 2 cloves of garlic
- 1 tsp Worcestershire sauce
- 100 gr gherkin slices
- 75 gr grated mozzarella
- 50 gr grated cheddar cheese
- 2 tbsp sesame seeds
- 400 g iceberg lettuce
- salt and pepper to taste

Sauce:

- 50 ml of mayonnaise
- 100 ml Greek yogurt, 10% fat
- 2 tsp mustard
- 1/2 tsp Worcestershire sauce
- 1 tbsp vinegar

- 1/2 tsp paprika
- 1/2 tsp onion powder
- 1/4 tsp garlic powder

PREPARATION METHOD

1. Preheat the convection oven to 180 degrees. Then cut the onion into small pieces and overwhelm the cloves of garlic. Heat a tablespoon of oil in a large frying pan. Add the onion, garlic, ground beef, Worcestershire sauce, salt, and pepper to the pan. Fry the minced meat whilst stirring and let the extra moisture drain out.

2. Meanwhile, make the Big Mac sauce by using blending all of the sauce substances in a bowl. Then spoon the minced meat right into a big bowl and add the grated mozzarella and half of the Big Mac sauce. Mix this nicely and then placed it in a greased oven dish.

3. Divide the pickle slices over the dish and sprinkle with the cheddar cheese and sesame seeds. Bake the Big Mac casserole for 15-20 minutes within the preheated oven. Divide the sliced iceberg lettuce over 4 plates and serve with the minced meat and the ultimate Big Mac sauce. Enjoy your meal!

NUTRITIONAL VALUES

Serving Size: 1/4 of the dish
Calories: 490
Fat: 35.9

Carbohydrates: 6.5
Proteins: 35.

Stuffed peppers with minced meat

Cooking time: 10 mins
Total time: 30 mins

INGREDIENTS

- 300 gr of lean ground beef
- 1 tbsp olive oil
- 1/2 onion
- 1 clove of garlic
- 1/2 tsp chili powder
- 1/2 tsp cumin powder
- 100 gr tomato cubes
- 60 gr grated cheese
- 2 large red peppers
- optional: crème fraîche

PREPARATION METHOD

1. Preheat the oven to 2 hundred degree. Clean the peppers and get rid of the tops and seeds. Place the peppers on a greased baking dish and drizzle with a touch of olive oil.
2. Cut the onion into small pieces and weigh down the garlic. Heat a tablespoon of olive oil and upload the chopped onion and beaten garlic. Fry for two mins, till the onion begins to discolor. Then add the minced meat and fry it until performed. Then upload the herbs and diced tomatoes and permit them to simmer for 5-10 minutes.
3. Remove the pan from the warmth and stir in 1/2 of the grated cheese. Fill the peppers with the minced meat mixture and garnish with a little cheese. Bake the crammed peppers within the preheated oven for 20 minutes. Serve the filled peppers with a clean salad and crème fraîche. Enjoy your meal!

NUTRITIONAL VALUES

Serving Size: 1 stuffed bell pepper
Calories: 474
Fats: 30.6
Carbohydrates: 9.6
Fiber: 2.9
Proteins: 39.4

Asparagus quiche with ham

Cooking time: 30 mins
Total time: 40 mins

INGREDIENTS

- 5 eggs
- 200 gr green asparagus (tips)
- 200 gr crème fraîche
- 125 gr ham cubes
- 100 gr cherry tomatoes
- 75 gr grated cheese
- 1 onion
- 1 tbsp olive oil
- pinch of nutmeg
- salt and pepper to taste

PREPARATION METHOD

1. Preheat the oven to 200 degree. Remove the bottom of the asparagus and bring a pan of water to a boil. Add the asparagus to the pan and prepare dinner till al dente for 4-eight minutes.
2. In the period in-between cut the onion into rings and the cherry tomatoes in 1/2. Add the onions to a frying pan with olive oil and fry for two minutes, till the onion starts to discolor. Then upload the ham cubes and fry them in short.
3. Grease a quiche tin with a bit of olive oil and set aside. Then, in a big bowl, integrate the eggs, crème fraîche, grated cheese, salt, pepper, and nutmeg. Add the fried onion and ham cubes and blend well once more.
4. Divide the cooked asparagus and halved cherry tomatoes over the quiche tin and pour the egg aggregate over it. Bake the asparagus quiche for 30-35 minutes inside the preheated oven. Cut the quiche into four pieces after baking. Enjoy your meal!

NUTRITIONAL VALUES .

Serving Size: 1/4 of the quiche
Calories: 360
Fat: 28.9

Carbohydrates: 5.2
Proteins: 19.2

Zucchini ravioli with spinach

Cooking time: 15 mins
Total time: 25 mins

INGREDIENTS

- 2 courgettes
- 75 gr spinach
- 1 small onion
- 1 clove of garlic
- dash of olive oil
- 250 gr ricotta cheese
- handful of fresh basil, finely chopped
- salt and pepper to taste
- 250 gr tomato sauce
- 50 gr grated mozzarella

PREPARATION METHOD.

1. Heat the convection oven to 220 ranges. Cut off the ends of the courgettes on a massive cutting board. Then take a potato peeler or cheese slicer and cut the zucchini into skinny slices. Place the slices on a plate and set them aside.
2. Cut the onion into small pieces and squeeze the garlic. Heat a drizzle of olive oil in a frying pan and upload the chopped onion and overwhelmed garlic. Fry for 2 mins, till the onion starts off evolved to discolor.
3. Finely chop the spinach and add it to the frying pan. Fry the spinach for 3 minutes, till the moisture has dissolved. Then integrate the ricotta, basil, salt, and pepper in a bowl. Add the fried and onion spinach to the bowl and blend properly with the ricotta.
4. Now take the plate with the zucchini slices. To shape the ravioli, first region 2 slices horizontally on a plate and 2 slices vertically on top. Spoon a tablespoon of the ricotta aggregate onto the middle of the 4 slices. Now first fold the lowest two slices up to the middle, secondly proper slices towards the middle, thirdly the left slices after the center and in the end the pinnacle slices after her the center. Flip the zucchini ravioli and region on a shelf. Repeat this step till all your zucchini slices are gone.
5. Pour the tomato sauce into a massive oven dish and punctiliously region the zucchini ravioli in the oven dish with the use of a cheese slicer or cake server. Sprinkle the ravioli with grated mozzarella and bake the oven dish for 15-20 mins inside the preheated oven. After baking, divide the dish into 3 portions. Enjoy your meal!

NUTRITIONAL VALUES

Serving Size: 1/3 of the dish
Calories: 275
Fat: 17.3

Carbohydrates: 13.1
Proteins: 16.1

11. Oven dish with leek and minced meat

Cooking time: 30 mins
Total time: 40 mins

INGREDIENTS

- 500 gr of lean ground beef
- 3 stalks of leek (400 gr)
- 1 small onion
- 1 clove of garlic
- dash of olive oil
- 2 tsp curry powder
- 1/2 tsp onion powder
- 1 cauliflower (500 g)
- 1 vegetable stock cube
- 50 gr cream cheese
- pinch of nutmeg
- 80 gr grated cheese
- salt and pepper to taste
- optional: fresh parsley

PREPARATION METHOD

1. Cut the onion into small pieces and crush the garlic. In a large skillet, warmth a drizzle of olive oil over medium warmness. Add the onion and garlic and fry until the onion starts to discolor. Then upload the minced meat, curry powder, onion powder, salt, and pepper. Fry the minced meat and reduce the leek into jewelry within the period in-between. Add the sliced leek and fry for 5 minutes. Turn off the warmth and let the excess fats drain in the pan.

2. Preheat the oven to a hundred and eighty degree Then reduce the cauliflower into florets on a huge cutting board. Add the cauliflower and the stock cube to a saucepan and fill it with water. Bring the water to a boil and cook dinner the cauliflower for about 12 minutes till smooth.

3. After cooking, pour the contents of the pan into a colander and let the water drain well. Pat the cauliflower florets dry with a paper towel and placed them back within the pan. Add the cream cheese and season with a pinch of nutmeg, salt, and pepper. Then puree the cauliflower with a hand blender right into a puree.

4. Spoon the minced meat combination into an oven dish and spoon over the cauliflower puree. Sprinkle the casserole with cheese and garnish with fresh parsley if preferred. Bake the oven dish with leek and minced meat for approx. 25 minutes inside the preheated oven.

NUTRITIONAL VALUES

Serving Size: 1/4 of the dish
Calories: 412
Fats: 34.6

Carbohydrates: 9.6
Fiber: 5.0
Proteins: 25.6

Low-carbohydrate chili con carne

Cooking time: 40 mins
Total time: 50 mins

INGREDIENTS

- 500 gr (lean) ground beef
- 1 onion
- 1 green pepper
- dash of olive oil
- 1 jalapeño pepper
- 1 clove of garlic, finely crushed
- 2 tbsp tomato paste
- 1 beef stock cube
- 450 ml of water
- 400 gr canned tomatoes
- 1 - 2 tsp chili powder or to taste
- 1 tsp cumin powder

- optional: grated cheddar and sour cream

PREPARATION METHOD

1. On a big reducing board, cut the onion, green pepper into small portions. Heat the olive oil in a large stockpot or frying pan. Add the minced meat, chopped onion, and bell pepper to the pan and fry it inside five mins while stirring. Then drain the excess fat from the pan.
2. Then reduce the jalapeño into small portions and cast off the seeds. Add the jalapeño, crushed garlic, diced tomatoes, tomato paste, stock cube, water, and herbs to the pan. Bring this to the boil and let it simmer for an approximate half-hour over a low warmness, till the sauce has thickened.
3. Divide the low-carb chili over four bowls and serve with a handful of grated cheddar and bitter cream if desired. Enjoy your meal!

NUTRITIONAL VALUES

Serving Size: 1 bowl (1/4)
Calories: 367
Fat: 24.9

Carbohydrates: 7.3
Proteins: 26.6

Caesar salad with chicken

Cooking time: 20 mins
Total time: 30 mins

INGREDIENTS

Salad:

- 1 chicken fillet
- 100 gr chopped romaine lettuce
- 1 slice of (fried) bacon
- 1/4 cucumber
- handful of cherry tomatoes
- 1/2 avocado
- 1 tbsp grated parmesan cheese
- 1/4 tsp paprika powder
- oregano to taste
- salt and pepper to taste

Caesar Dressing:

- 1 tbsp mayonnaise
- 1 tsp mustard
- 1/2 tsp lemon juice
- 1/2 tbsp grated parmesan cheese
- optional: Worcestershire sauce

PREPARATION METHOD

1. Preheat the oven to one hundred eighty degree. Season the chook breast with paprika, oregano, salt, and pepper. Place the chicken breast on a baking tray coated with parchment paper. Bake the chicken breast for 15-20 minutes in the preheated oven.
2. Meanwhile cut the cucumber into slices, the avocado into strips, and the cherry tomatoes in half. Then, in a huge bowl, integrate the romaine lettuce, cucumber, avocado, cherry tomatoes, and bacon. Then make the dressing by using mixing the mayonnaise, mustard, lemon juice, grated cheese, and Worcestershire sauce in a small bowl.
3. Remove the hen breast from the oven and reduce it into strips or cubes. Serve the Caesar salad with the dressing and sprinkle the salad with a touch of grated cheese if preferred. Enjoy your meal!

NUTRITIONAL VALUES

Serving Size: 1 portion
Calories: 553
Fats: 36.1

Carbohydrates: 5.0
Fiber: 6.3
Proteins: 47.8

Oven dish with zucchini and chicken

Cooking time: 30 mins
Total time: 40 mins

INGREDIENTS

- 300 gr chicken cubes
- 350 gr mushrooms
- 3 medium zucchini
- 1/2 onion
- 2 tbsp olive oil
- 250 whipped cream
- 50 ml of water
- 1/2 cube of chicken stock
- 85 gr grated Gruyere cheese
- salt and pepper to taste
- optional: arrowroot or cornstarch

PREPARATION METHOD

1. Preheat the convection oven to a hundred ninety degrees. Cut the mushrooms into slices, the courgettes into cubes, and the onion into small portions on a massive reducing board. Then heat a tablespoon of olive oil in a massive frying pan and add the mushrooms and onion. Bake for four-6 minutes, till onion starts to discolor. Then add the zucchini cubes and fry for eight-10 minutes.
2. After baking, permit it to drain the excess moisture from the pan. Spoon the fried greens into a bowl and easy the pan. Return the pan to heat and add a tbsp olive oil. Then add the hen cubes to the pan and season with salt and pepper. Fry the chicken cubes for approximately 5 minutes until golden brown and finished.
3. After cooking, add the cubes to the bowl with the veggies and then get a large saucepan. Place the saucepan on a low warmness and pour the whipped cream into the pan. Add the hen stock and water to the pan and produce to the boil. Let it simmer for 10 minutes until the sauce has thickened. Then upload half of the Gruyere cheese to the pan and gently stir it into the sauce. If the sauce is just too skinny, you can upload a teaspoon of arrowroot or cornstarch if essential.
4. Now drain the extra liquid from the bowl with the veggies and chicken. Then divide the fried vegetables and hen cubes over an oven dish and season with salt and pepper. Pour the cheese sauce over the greens and hen and ultimately sprinkle the relaxation of the Gruyere cheese over the dish. Bake the oven dish for 20-25 mins within the preheated oven. After baking, divide into four portions and enjoy!

NUTRITIONAL VALUES

Serving Size: 1/4 of the dish
Calories: 494
Fats: 35.1

Carbohydrates: 12.6
Proteins: 30.9

Tandoori chicken with broccoli rice

Cooking time: 35 mins
Total time: 105 mins

INGREDIENTS

- 300 gr chicken cubes
- 150 gr Greek yogurt, 10% fat
- 2 cm ginger, grated
- 1 clove of garlic, crushed
- 1/2 tsp cinnamon
- 1/2 tsp cayenne pepper
- 1 tsp turmeric
- 1/2 tsp ground coriander
- 1 tsp cumin powder
- 2 tbsp tomato paste
- salt and pepper to taste
- 2 tbsp olive oil
- 1 onion
- 1/2 red bell pepper
- 400 gr broccoli rice

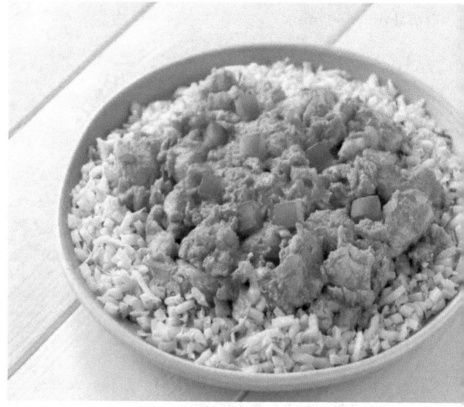

- optional: crème fraîche

PREPARATION METHOD

1. In a big bowl, integrate the hen cubes, grated ginger, crushed garlic, Greek yogurt, cinnamon, cayenne pepper, turmeric, cilantro, cumin powder, tomato paste, salt, and pepper. Cover the bowl or with a dangle movie and let the marinade relax for at least 1 hour inside the refrigerator.
2. Cut the onion and purple pepper into small portions and warm a tablespoon of olive oil in a frying pan. Add the sliced onion and bell pepper to the pan and sauté till the onion starts to discolor. Then add the marinated bird and the marinade to the pan and decrease the heat to low. Bake the bird for about 15-20 mins.
3. When the chook is cooked, take another frying pan and warm a tbsp olive oil in it. Add the broccoli rice to the pan and wok it within 2-3 minutes. Divide the broccoli rice and tandoori bird between two plates. Serve with a part of crème fraîche if desired. Enjoy your meal!

NUTRITIONAL VALUES

Serving size: 1/2 of the total
Calories: 435
Fat: 21.3

Carbohydrates: 9.8
Fiber: 7.5
Proteins: 46.5

Low-carbohydrate quesadilla

Cooking time: 20 mins
Total time: 30 mins

INGREDIENTS

- 150 gr chicken cubes
- 2 tbsp olive oil
- 1/2 tbsp taco seasoning
- 1/4 red bell pepper
- 1/2 onion
- 2 low- carb wraps from Atkins
- 50 gr grated cheddar or Mexican cheese
- optional: sour cream or salsa

PREPARATION METHOD

1. Heat a tablespoon of olive oil in a big frying pan. Add the chook cubes to the pan and fry for about five mins at the same time as stirring. Meanwhile, reduce the onion and bell pepper into small portions.
2. When the chook is cooked, add the chopped onion, bell pepper, and taco seasoning to the pan and fry for three to five minutes. Then scoop the contents of the pan right into a bowl and easy the pan.
3. Now take the wraps and rub one side of each wrap with a touch of olive oil. Place a wrap oil-aspect down on a board and sprinkle half of the grated cheese at the wrap. Then spoon the chook filling on the wrap and sprinkle the relaxation of the cheese on the pinnacle. Finally, place the opposite tortilla oil-facet up on top of the filled wrap.
4. Heat the skillet over medium heat and add the stuffed quesadilla to the pan. Put the lid on the pan and bake the quesadilla for two-4 mins. Then gently turn the quesadilla with a spatula or cheese slicer and bake for another 2 mins.
5. Remove the quesadilla from the pan after baking and cut into four portions. Divide the 4 pieces over 2 plates and serve with salsa or bitter cream if favored. Enjoy your meal!

NUTRITIONAL VALUES

Serving Size: 1/2 quesadilla
Calories: 413
Fats: 23.6
Carbohydrates: 8.0

Fiber: 11.7
Proteins: 33.6

Cauliflower risotto with mushrooms

Cooking time: 15 mins
Total time: 25 mins

INGREDIENTS

- 300 g cauliflower rice
- 225 gr (chestnut) mushrooms
- 1 small onion
- 1 small clove of garlic, crushed
- 2 tbsp olive oil
- 60 ml of water
- 1/4 chicken stock cube
- 30 g grated parmesan cheese
- 30 gr grated mozzarella
- 1 tbsp parsley, finely chopped
- salt and pepper to taste

PREPARATION METHOD

1. Cut the onion into small portions and the mushrooms into slices on a reducing board. Then warmness a tablespoon of olive oil in a big frying pan. Add the mushrooms to the pan and fry it within approx. 5 minutes. Remove the mushrooms from the pan after frying and clean the pan.
2. Take the pan and upload some other tbsp olive oil. Then add the sliced onion and pressed garlic to the pan and fry it until the onion starts off evolved to discolor. Add the cauliflower rice, mushrooms, water, inventory dice, salt, and pepper to the pan and cook dinner without a lid for 4 mins.
3. Remove the pan from the warmth and allow the extra liquid to drain. Then add the grated mozzarella and parmesan cheese and stir this through the cauliflower risotto. Divide the risotto among two plates and serve with clean parsley.

NUTRITIONAL VALUES

Serving Size: 1/2 of the risotto
Calories: 253
Fats: 17.7
Carbohydrates: 6.3

Fiber: 5.0
Proteins: 14.7

Chicory dish with minced meat

Cooking time: 35 mins
Total time: 45 mins

INGREDIENTS

- 300 gr (lean) ground beef
- 1 large onion
- 1 tbsp olive oil
- 500 gr chicory
- 1 red pepper
- 100 gr smoked ham
- 100 gr of grated cheese
- 75 gr cream cheese
- 150 ml of cooking cream
- 1 tbsp mustard
- 50 gr grated mozzarella
- salt and pepper to taste
- optional: spring onion

PREPARATION METHOD

1. Preheat the oven to 190 degrees. Cut the onion and bell pepper into small portions on a reducing board. Then take the chicory, dispose of the outer leaves and the ends. Cut each stump in 1/2 and cast off the bitter middle with a pointy knife. Finally, reduce the chicory into smaller pieces.

2. Heat a tablespoon of olive oil in a huge frying pan and add the sliced onion. Saute the onion until it starts off evolved to discolor, then upload the floor beef. Fry the minced meat for approximately three-five mins after which upload the chopped bell pepper and chicory. Fry the greens for five minutes after which permit the excess liquid to drain in the pan. Then reduce the smoked ham into small pieces and add this to the minced meat and vegetables within the pan.

3. Now take a small saucepan and warm the cooking cream, cream cheese, and grated cheese in it. Reduce warmth and convey to a boil. Cook the cheese sauce until the grated cheese within the pan has melted. Then put off the pan from the warmth and add the mustard whilst stirring.

4. Divide the minced meat combination over an oven dish and season with salt and pepper. Then pour the cheese sauce over the minced meat aggregate and sprinkle with the grated mozzarella. Bake the chicory dish for 25-30 minutes within the preheated oven. After baking, garnish the chicory dish with chopped spring onion.

NUTRITIONAL VALUES

| Serving Size: 1/4 of the dish | Fat: 33.5 | Fiber: 1.8 |
| Calories: 473 | Carbohydrates: 8.9 | Proteins: 33.9 |

Low-carbohydrate rendang

Cooking time: 15 mins
Total time: 130 mins

INGREDIENTS

- 800 gr ribs
- 2 onions
- 1 red pepper
- 2 - 3 cloves of garlic
- fresh ginger (3 cm)
- 1 tsp laos
- 2 tsp turmeric
- 1 tsp cumin powder
- 1 tsp cilantro, ground
- 2 stems of lemongrass
- 1/2 stock cube
- 1 bay leaf
- 2 tbsp olive oil
- 1 tbsp tomato paste

- 400 ml canned coconut milk

PREPARATION METHOD

1. Cut the ribs into small cubes and season with salt and pepper. Chop the onion, press the garlic and reduce the purple pepper and ginger into small pieces.
2. Heat a dash of olive oil in a casserole and fry the portions of meat all around brown. Add the chopped onion, garlic, and crimson pepper to the pan and fry for 2 minutes. Then add the ginger and the rest of the spices to the pan and cook for a minute.
3. Meanwhile, overwhelm the lemongrass stems. You do this by tapping the stems a few times with the blunt side of a knife. Then add the stems along with the coconut milk, tomato paste, inventory dice, and bay leaf to the pan.
4. Lower the heat and simmer lightly for two hours with the lid on the pan. Stir the pan from time to time to save the meat from burning. After 2 hours, take away the lid and simmer the rendang for a further 10-15 mins to thicken the sauce.
5. When the rendang is executed, cast off the bay leaf and lemongrass stems from the pan. Divide the rendang over four plates and serve with a part of cauliflower rice and green beans if favored.

NUTRITIONAL VALUES

Serving size: 1/4 of the total
Calories: 537
Fats: 40.0

Carbohydrates: 4.2
Proteins: 39.6

Butter chicken with cauliflower rice

Cooking time: 35 mins
Total time: 65 mins

INGREDIENTS

Marinade:

- 600 gr chicken fillet cubes
- 125 gr Greek yogurt, 10% fat
- 2 tsp garam masala
- 1 tsp turmeric
- 1 tsp chili powder
- 1 tsp cumin powder
- 2 cloves of garlic, finely crushed
- 1 tbsp fresh ginger, grated
- salt and pepper to taste

Curry:

- tbsp olive oil
- 2 tbsp ghee or unsalted butter
- 1 onion
- 1 clove of garlic, finely crushed
- 1 tbsp fresh ginger, grated

- 1 tsp garam masala
- 400 gr tomato pulp (Mutti)
- 150 ml of whipped cream
- 1/2 tsp salt or to taste
- 600 gr cauliflower rice

PREPARATION METHOD

1. In a bowl, blend the total-fats yogurt with the marinade herbs, overwhelmed garlic, and grated ginger. Add the bird fillet cubes and stir well via the marinade. Put the chicken breast cubes within the fridge and permit the marinade to soak for a minimum of 1 hour.

2. Heat 2 tbsp olive oil in a big skillet. Remove the bird breast cubes from the marinade and add the cubes to the pan. Fry the chicken fillet cubes for approximately 4-6 mins until golden brown. Spoon the fried chook breast cubes briefly onto a plate and smooth the pan.

3. Cut the onion into small portions on a reducing board and squeeze a clove of garlic. Then heat 2 tbsp ghee or butter in the easy frying pan. Add the sliced onion and beaten garlic and saute till it starts to discolor for approximately three mins. Then upload the grated ginger and garam masala and fry it in short. Then upload the tomato pulp and half of the tsp salt to the pan. Reduce heat and allow the sauce to simmer for 10 minutes.

4. After simmering, add the whipped cream and fried chicken breast cubes to the sauce and simmer for another 10 minutes, until the chook is cooked and the sauce has thickened. Meanwhile, fry the cauliflower rice in another frying pan for 2-three mins.

5. Divide the cauliflower rice and butter bird among 4 plates and garnish with clean parsley or coriander. Enjoy your meal!

NUTRITIONAL VALUES

Serving Size: 1/4 of the curry

Calories: 481

Fat: 28.0

Carbohydrates: 11.8

Proteins: 42.3

Low-carbohydrate quiche lorraine

Cooking time: 25 mins
Total time: 45 mins

INGREDIENTS

- 5 eggs (M)
- 200 gr creme fraiche
- 2 tbsp olive oil
- 1 onion
- 1 leek
- 200 gr bacon strips
- 100 gr grated Gruyère cheese
- pinch of nutmeg
- salt and pepper to taste
- optional: spring onion, sliced

PREPARATION METHOD

1. Preheat the oven to two hundred ranges. Then cut the onion and leek into small pieces. Heat a tablespoon of olive oil in a frying pan and fry the chopped leek and onion. Put the fried onion and leek in a field and ease the frying pan.
2. Now fry the bacon cubes inside the frying pan until golden brown. After baking, drain the bacon cubes on a paper towel. Then beat the eggs with the crème fraîche. Then add the grated Gruyere cheese and season with the nutmeg, salt, and pepper.
3. Grease a quiche tin with a touch of oil or butter. Then divide the fried bacon cubes, onion, and leek over the quiche pan and pour the egg combination over it. Bake the quiche Lorraine for 30-35 minutes in the preheated oven. After baking, divide the quiche into four portions and serve with chopped spring onion if favored. Enjoy your meal!

NUTRITIONAL VALUES

Serving Size: 1/4 of the quiche
Calories: 483
Fats: 42.1

Carbohydrates: 3.3
Proteins: 22.3

Salad with smoked salmon and avocado

Cooking time: 10 mins
Total time: 10 mins

INGREDIENTS

Salad:

- 125 gr warm smoked salmon fillet
- 100 gr radish
- 1 avocado
- 1/2 red onion
- 75 gr arugula salad mix
- optional: cucumber

Dill dressing:

- 30 ml mayonnaise or Greek yogurt
- 1 tbsp olive oil
- 1/2 tbsp apple cider vinegar
- 1/2 tbsp mustard
- 1 tbsp fresh or dried dill
- salt and pepper to taste
- optional: 1 clove of garlic, crushed

PREPARATION METHOD

Cut the radishes into slices, the avocado into portions, and the onions into earrings on a massive board. Then divide the sliced veggies and arugula salad blend over plates. Cut the salmon steak into small pieces and heat the pieces in brief in the microwave. You also can serve the salmon pieces cold.

Meanwhile, make the dressing by way of whipping all elements together in a bowl with a whisk. Divide the heated salmon pieces between the 2 plates and drizzle the salad with the dill dressing. Enjoy your meal!

Nutritional values

Serving Size: 1/2 of the salad

Calories: 405

Fat: 34.5

Carbohydrates: 5.5

Fiber: 2.5

Proteins: 16.2

Courgetti with meatballs

Cooking time: 15 mins
Total time: 35 mins

INGREDIENTS

Meatballs:

- 300 gr ground beef
- 1 egg (M)
- 1/2 onion
- 1 small clove of garlic
- 1 tbsp almond flour
- 2 tbsp olive oil
- 20 gr grated parmigiano reggiano
- 1/2 tsp Italian herbs
- salt and pepper to taste

Courgetti:

- 400 gr zucchini spaghetti
- 1 can of tomato pulp or diced tomatoes (400 gr)
- 1 tbsp tomato paste
- 1/2 onion

- 1 clove of garlic
- 1/2 bouillion cube
- 125 ml of water
- 1 tsp Italian herbs
- 1 bay leaf
- 50 gr arugula

PREPARATION METHOD

1. Cut the onions into small pieces and crush the garlic with a garlic press. Then, in a massive bowl, integrate the floor red meat, onion, garlic, grated Parmigiano Reggiano, and Italian herbs. Beat the egg and upload it to the bowl at the side of the almond flour and blend properly once more.
2. Shape the minced meat into 9 small meatballs. Heat a tablespoon of olive oil or butter in a big frying pan and fry the meatballs over low heat for about 10 mins. After baking, an area the balls on a plate and smooth the frying pan.
3. Heat a tablespoon of olive oil inside the identical frying pan and upload the onion and garlic. Saute until the onion and garlic begin to discolor. Fry the tomato paste in brief for a minute after which add the tomato pulp, Italian herbs, inventory cube, water, and the bay leaf. Bring to a boil and simmer the tomato sauce over low warmth for 15-20 minutes.
4. After simmering, upload the meatballs and heat them briefly in the sauce. Then take a wok pan and wok the zucchini spaghetti in it for two minutes. Divide the spaghetti and tomato sauce with meatballs amongst 3 plates. Serve the spaghetti with the arugula and garnish with Parmigiano Reggiano. Enjoy your meal

NUTRITIONAL VALUES

Serving size: 1/3 of the total
Calories: 395
Fats: 22.9

Carbohydrates: 14.6
Proteins: 30.8

Oven dish with chicken and vegetables

Cooking time: 10 mins
Total time: 40 mins

INGREDIENTS

- 300 gr chicken fillet cubes
- 1/2 onion
- 2 tbsp olive oil
- 250 gr mushrooms
- 1 broccoli
- 400 gr of cauliflower rice
- 2 large eggs
- 135 gr herb cream cheese
- 50 gr grated mozzarella
- 50 gr grated mature cheese
- salt and pepper to taste

PREPARATION METHOD

1. Preheat the oven to 180 degree. Add a tablespoon of olive oil to a massive skillet and warm it over medium warmth. Then sprinkle the chook breast cubes with salt and pepper or your favorite spice blend. Add the bird breast cubes to the frying pan and fry for about 5 minutes until brown and done. Put the fried hen in a bowl and ease the pan.

2. Then reduce the onion and mushrooms into small pieces. Take the easy skillet and upload a tablespoon of olive oil to the pan. When the olive oil is heat, add the chopped onions and fry them until they start to colorate. Then add the mushrooms and fry them for 2 minutes at the same time as stirring. Add the chicken to the pan and turn off the heat.

3. Meanwhile cut the broccoli into small florets and cook for five mins in a pan full of boiling water. After cooking, drain the water and add the florets to the pan with the chicken. Then take a frying pan and stir the cauliflower rice al dente within 2 minutes. Also, upload the cauliflower rice to the pan with the bird after baking.

4. Then beat the eggs in a large bowl with a whisk. Add the herb cream cheese and blend until lumps are gone. Finally, add the grated mature cheese to the bowl and whisk it in brief via the egg mixture.

5. Add the egg mixture to the pan with the chook and veggies and mix nicely. Spoon the bird and vegetables right into a large baking dish and sprinkle with the grated mozzarella. Bake the casserole for 25-30 minutes inside the preheated oven. Divide into four quantities after baking. Enjoy your meal!

NUTRITIONAL VALUES

Serving Size: 1/4 of the dish

Calories: 375

Fats: 21.1

Carbohydrates: 6.8

Fiber: 3.9

Proteins: 36.8

Courgetti carbonara

INGREDIENTS

- 400 gr zucchini spaghetti
- 100 gr bacon strips
- 125 gr mushrooms
- 125 ml of whipped cream
- 40 g grated parmesan cheese
- 1 clove of garlic
- 1/2 onion
- optional: handful of arugula

PREPARATION METHOD

1. Cut the onion and mushrooms into small pieces on a reducing board and crush the garlic with a garlic press. Then pour a tablespoon of olive oil into a frying pan and fry the onion and garlic for approximately 2 minutes, until the onion starts to discolor.
2. Then upload the mushrooms and bacon bits to the frying pan and fry for four-five mins, until the bacon is crispy. Allow the excess moisture to drain from the pan whilst baking. Finally, upload the whipped cream and grated parmesan cheese to the pan while stirring, cook dinner for 2 mins and turn off the warmth whilst the whole lot is well blended.
3. Meanwhile, fry the zucchini spaghetti in another frying pan within 2 mins. After baking, drain the excess liquid and then stir the spaghetti into the carbonara sauce. Divide into 2 quantities and enjoy!

NUTRITIONAL VALUES

Serving size: 1/2 of the total
Calories: 502
Fats: 39.9

Carbohydrates: 13.4
Fiber: 2.3
Proteins: 21.9

LUNCH

Omelette with baby spinach

Cooking time: 10 mins
Total time: 25 mins

INGREDIENTS

- 2 - 3 medium eggs
- 30 g baby spinach, cut into pieces
- 10 gr Parmesan cheese, grated
- 1/4 tsp onion powder
- 1/8 tsp nutmeg
- salt and pepper to taste

PREPARATION METHOD

1. In a massive bowl, beat the eggs and add the spinach and Parmesan cheese whilst stirring. Season with onion powder, nutmeg, salt, and pepper.
2. Grease a small skillet with butter or oil and warm the pan over medium warmth. Add the egg aggregate to the pan and cook dinner the omelet on one aspect for approximately 3 minutes. Then turn the omelet with a spatula and fry for every other three minutes. Now decrease the heat and cook for any other 2 minutes. Enjoy your meal!

NUTRITIONAL VALUES

Serving Size: 1 omelet
Calories: 186
Fats: 12.7

Carbohydrates: 2.9
Proteins: 17.0

Savory ham cheese muffins

Cooking time: 10 mins
Total time: 35 mins

INGREDIENTS

- 125 gr ham cubes
- 125 gr grated cheese
- 4 medium eggs
- 45 gr green pepper
- 1 celery stalk
- 1 tbsp chives, finely chopped
- 1 tbsp parsley, finely chopped
- 1/4 tsp onion powder
- 1/4 tsp pepper

PREPARATION METHOD

1. Preheat the oven to one hundred eighty degrees. Cut the bell pepper and celery into small pieces on a huge slicing board. Then grind the ham in a food processor. Then mix all components in a huge bowl.
2. Divide the mixture from the bowl over the 6 muffin cups. Place the aluminum muffin cases on an oven rack lined with parchment paper. Bake the cakes inside the preheated oven for approximately 25-half-hour until golden brown. Let the truffles cool at the rack for 10 mins. Remove the muffins from the tin and serve.

NUTRITIONAL VALUES

Serving Size: 1 muffin
Calories: 157
Fat: 11.3
Carbohydrates: 1.8
Proteins: 11.7

Cheese waffles

Cooking time: 18 mins
Total time: 28 mins

INGREDIENTS

- 100 g cauliflower, finely ground
- 110 gr grated mozzarella cheese, finely ground
- 35 gr grated Parmesan cheese
- 2 medium eggs
- 1 tbsp chives
- 1 tsp garlic powder
- 1 tsp onion powder
- 1/2 tsp black pepper

PREPARATION METHOD

1. In a large bowl, mix all elements well. Then warmth the waffle iron. Place 1/4 cup of the batter inside the waffle iron. Bake the waffles for 4 to 6 mins.
2. If the waffles still keep on with the iron after 6 mins, let them bake for a while. Repeat this till you have baked four waffles. Let the waffles cool on a plate and positioned the waffles you may not consume inside the fridge.

NUTRITIONAL VALUES

Serving Size: 1 wafer
Calories: 160
Fats: 11.2
Carbohydrates: 1.7
Proteins: 13.2

Cream cheese pancakes

Cooking time: 10 mins
Total time: 15 mins

INGREDIENTS

- 55 gr cream cheese
- 2 medium eggs
- 1/2 tsp cinnamon
- stevia or erythritol to taste

PREPARATION METHOD

1. Place all elements in a blender or food processor. Turn on the blender and mix until clean. After blending permit the batter to rest outdoor in the fridge for 2 mins.
2. Heat a greased skillet over medium heat. You can select to bake one big pancake or two to 3 small ones. Add the butter and fry the pancake till bubbles seem on the top of the pancake and the rims are dry. Then turn the pancake and bake it for every other 1 minute

NUTRITIONAL VALUES

Serving Size: 1 large pancake
Calories: 344
Fats: 29.1
Carbohydrates: 2.5
Proteins: 17.2

Savory egg muffins

Cooking time: 35 mins　　　　　　　　　**Total time: 45 mins**

INGREDIENTS

- 6 medium eggs
- 100 gr of lean ground beef
- 1 small onion
- 1/2 red bell pepper
- handful of fresh spinach
- 1 clove of garlic, finely crushed
- 1 tbsp coconut oil
- 2 tsp tomato paste
- 1/2 tsp finely ground cumin
- salt and pepper to taste

PREPARATION METHOD

1. Preheat the oven to 180 ° C and grease a muffin tin with 6 ramekins with a bit of coconut oil. Then beat the eggs in a bowl and mix in the tomato puree, salt, and pepper.
2. Melt a tablespoon of coconut oil in a massive frying pan over medium warmness and sauté the onion in it. Add the finely beaten garlic, minced meat, and cumin and fry for 5-10 mins on low warmth. Finally, add the bell pepper and spinach and fry it briefly.
3. Remove the frying pan from the warmth and upload the minced meat aggregate to the egg combination and stir nicely. Then pour the egg aggregate into the muffin tin and bake the egg desserts for 15-25 mins in the preheated oven or until a skewer comes out clean. Enjoy your meal!

NUTRITIONAL VALUES

Serving Size: 1 muffin　　　　　　Fat: 8.2　　　　　　　　　　Proteins: 9.4

Calories: 153　　　　　　　　　　Carbohydrates: 4.0

Low-carbohydrate rösti

Cooking time: 10 mins
Total time: 25 mins

INGREDIENTS

- 150 gr celeriac
- 1 tbsp olive oil
- 1 tbsp butter
- 15 g bacon, cut into small pieces
- 20 gr grated Parmesan cheese
- 1/2 tsp salt
- 1/8 tsp ground black pepper
- 1/4 tsp garlic powder
- handful of lamb's lettuce

PREPARATION METHOD

1. To start with, snatch the celeriac. Place the celeriac on a large slicing board and reduce the tuber in half. Then placed the celeriac flat jug on the board and thoroughly cut the skin away, till you're left with only the white flesh.
2. Then take a massive grater and grate a piece of the celeriac over a bowl. Grate the celeriac until you've got one hundred fifty grams of grated pulp. Add the parmesan cheese and the herbs and blend nicely.
3. Then heat the olive oil and butter in a frying pan over medium heat. Add the bacon and fry it crispy. Then add the celeriac mixture to the pan and press with the return of a big spoon at the aggregate to form a massive pancake.
4. Fry the rösti over medium to low warmth for approximately five mins. Until the bottom is golden brown and crispy. When the rösti is ready, take away the pain from the warmth and keep it the wrong way up over a plate, and punctiliously permit the rösti to fall. Serve the low-carb rösti warm or cold with a few lamb's lettuces!

NUTRITIONAL VALUES

Serving Size: 1 rösti
Calories: 332
Fats: 21.0

Carbohydrates: 8.3
Proteins: 13.3

Forest mushroom soup

Cooking time: 30 mins
Total time: 45 mins

INGREDIENTS

- 200 gr mushroom mix, sliced
- 125 ml of whipped cream
- 1 - 2 shallots
- 2 vegetable stock cubes
- 1 handful of fresh parsley
- optional: a drop of olive oil with truffle flavor

PREPARATION METHOD

1. Finely chop the shallots and fry them in a massive frying pan with olive oil. When the shallots flip color, add the mushroom mixture and fry briefly. Then take a huge stockpot and produce 1 liter of water to the boil.
2. When the water is boiling, upload the stock cubes to the stockpot and stir nicely. Add 3/4 of the baked mushroom mix, all of the shallots, and a hundred twenty-five ml of whipped cream to the stockpot and allow it to simmer for approximately 10 minutes on low heat.
3. After cooking for 10 minutes, puree the soup with a hand blender or blender. After blending, stir the last 1/four of the fried mushroom mixture into the soup and add chopped clean parsley. Enjoy your meal!

NUTRITIONAL VALUES

Serving Size: 1 bowl
Calories: 80
Fat: 7.4

Carbohydrates: 1.2
Proteins: 1.2

Low-carbohydrate Chinese chicken salad

Cooking time: 20 mins
Total time: 30 mins

INGREDIENTS

- 300 gr white cabbage, cut
- 200 gr Chinese cabbage, chopped
- 500 gr chicken fillet
- 4 cups of water
- 1/2 tsp garlic powder
- 1/2 tsp onion powder
- 1/4 tsp salt
- 20 ml soy sauce with less salt
- 3/4 cucumber
- 4 stalks of spring onion
- 150 gr radishes
- 2 tbsp sesame seeds
- bottle of Ready-to-use Oriental dressing (Jean Baton)
- 2 handfuls of fresh parsley, finely chopped

PREPARATION METHOD

In a big skillet, warm 4 cups of water, soy sauce, garlic powder, and onion powder. Stir briefly and then add the chook breasts to the pan. Bring the contents of the pan to the boil and simmer for 15-20 minutes with the lid at the pan.

Meanwhile, cut the cucumber, radishes, and spring onion into pieces. After 15-20 minutes of simmering, remove the skillet from the heat and place the chook breasts on a plate. Using a fork and knife, pull the chicken breasts aside into small portions.

Divide the Chinese cabbage, white cabbage, and chopped greens amongst 5 plates and area a little shredded chicken on top of every vegetable plate. Garnish with sesame seeds, parsley, and the Oriental salad dressing. Enjoy your meal!

NUTRITIONAL VALUES

Serving Size: 1/5
Calories: 187
Fats: 5.0

Carbohydrates: 6.0
Proteins: 26.2

Low-carbohydrate flaxseed buns

Cooking time: 15 mins
Total time: 25 mins

INGREDIENTS

- 80 gr linseed, broken
- 2 - 3 medium eggs
- 55 g grated Parmesan cheese

PREPARATION METHOD

1. Preheat the oven to one hundred eighty ° C. In a large bowl, mix all elements properly. Divide the batter into 6 equally sized dough balls.
2. Place a piece of baking paper on a baking tray and region the 6 balls of dough on it. Flatten the dough balls with the lower back of a spoon and shape them right into a round bun.
3. Bake the flaxseed buns inside the preheated oven for 10-12 mins. Let the rolls cool down after baking. Top the sandwiches along with your favored low-carbohydrate sandwich spread

NUTRITIONAL VALUES

Serving Size: 2 sandwiches
Calories: 223
Fat: 17.2
Carbohydrates: 2.3
Proteins: 15.1

Low-carbohydrate sushi

Cooking time: 15 mins
Total time: 15 mins

INGREDIENTS

- 2 nori sheets
- 1 ripe avocado
- 1/2 red bell pepper
- 1/4 carrot
- 1/4 cucumber
- 15 gr alfafa
- 1/4 red onion
- 1 tbsp sesame seeds
- soy sauce to taste

PREPARATION METHOD

1. Place the two nori sheets on a flat floor, worktop, or cutting board. Peel and reduce the avocado into cubes and put the cubes in a bowl. Then mash these cubes inside the bowl with a fork and set the bowl apart. Cut all of the greens into skinny strips and set this aside for a while.

2. Spread the avocado puree calmly on the lowest of both nori sheets. Carefully vicinity the thin strips of greens horizontally above the avocado puree on the nori sheets. Then take the lowest of the nori sheets and fold it over to the top of the filling, in the meantime keep the filling in an area with your hands and roll tightly until the end of the sheet. When you reach the end of the sheet, moist your index finger and roll the final piece. Then moisten your palms and rub the nori sheets. Wetting guarantees that the nori sheets stick collectively.

3. You can now cut the sushi rolls right into a preferred variety of portions with a pointy knife, but it is also viable to devour the roll like this. Garnish with the sesame seeds and serve with soy sauce. Enjoy your meal!

NUTRITIONAL VALUES

Serving Size: 1 roll
Calories: 201
Fats: 17.9

Carbohydrates: 6.0
Proteins: 4.1

Avocado tuna salad

Cooking time: 15 mins
Total time: 15 mins

INGREDIENTS

- 1 avocado
- lemon juice from 1 lemon
- 1/4 red onion, chopped
- 2 celery stalks, finely chopped
- 1 can of tuna in water
- salt and black pepper to taste

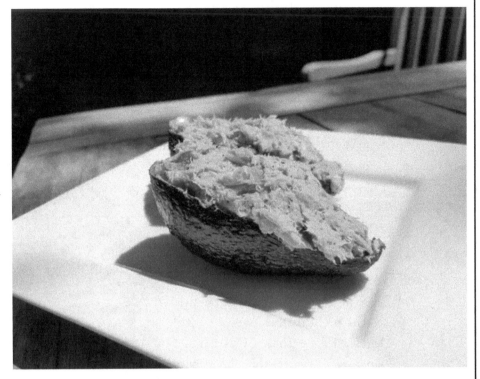

PREPARATION METHOD

1. Cut the avocado in 1/2 the usage of a knife. You do that by means of making a reduce lengthwise across the wick. Then turn the avocado along with your hands to loosen it. Then insert a pointy knife into the pit and lightly pull it out of the avocado 1/2.
2. Then spoon the pulp out of the avocado and keep the pores and skin. Mash the pulp in a bowl and add the red onion, celery, lemon juice, and herbs. Stir nicely after which add the drained tuna and blend well once more.
3. Return the avocado tuna salad to the avocado or location on a toasted low-carb sandwich. Enjoy your meal!

NUTRITIONAL VALUES

Serving Size: 1 portion
Calories: 304
Fat: 20.7

Carbohydrates: 4.4
Fiber: 6.9
Proteins: 21.6

Low-carbohydrate sandwich

Cooking time: 30 mins
Total time: 30 mins

INGREDIENTS

- 1 small cauliflower
- 1 large egg (L)
- 50 gr grated mozzarella
- 1/2 tsp salt
- 1/4 tsp black pepper
- extra spices to taste
- 1 tbsp butter
- 70 g spicy grated cheddar

PREPARATION METHOD

1. Place an oven rack in the oven after which preheat the oven to 220 degree. Take a sheet of parchment paper and grease the sheet with some olive oil.

2. Now take the small cauliflower and dispose of the leaves and black spots. Cut the cauliflower in 1/2 and cast off the stump. Cut what's left into small florets. Put the florets in a food processor or blender and turn it on until small rice grains form. Repeat this until you've got made rice from all of the florets. Are you short on time? Then use geared up-to-consume cauliflower rice

3. Heat and tbsp olive oil in a frying pan. Add the cauliflower rice to the pan and fry it inside four-five minutes. Let the rice calm down after baking and then add it to a smooth kitchen towel. Then wring out all of the moisture from the rice.

4. Place the dry rice in a large bowl and upload the grated mozzarella, egg, salt, and pepper. Add extra spices if favored. Mix the whole thing well inside the bowl with a whisk. Divide the batter over the baking paper and form 4 identical-sized squares. Bake the buns for 16 minutes till golden brown. Let cool for at least 10 mins after which cautiously remove the rolls from the baking paper with a cheese slicer.

5. Now grease one facet of each sandwich with butter. Heat a frying pan over medium heat and positioned the bun within the pan with the butter facet. Add shredded cheddar to the bun and put one bun on the pinnacle with the butter side up. Lower the heat and cook dinner for 2-4 minutes on every side, until the cheese has melted. Repeat with the alternative sandwiches!

NUTRITIONAL VALUES

Serving Size: 1 toasted sandwich
Calories: 343
Fats: 25.2

Carbohydrates: 6.0
Proteins: 21.3

Courgetti with chicken and pesto

Cooking time: 10 mins
Total time: 25 mins

INGREDIENTS

500 gr broccoli

- 400 gr chicken fillet à la minute
- 600 gr zucchini spaghetti
- 70 gr pesto alla Genovese
- 80 gr cherry tomatoes
- 30 gr pine nuts
- 75 gr arugula
- 50 gr grated Parmesan cheese
- 3 tbsp olive oil
- salt and pepper to taste
- optional: tablespoon of Crème fraîche

PREPARATION METHOD

1. Cut the broccoli into florets. Cook the broccoli in boiling water for 6-8 mins until tender. Meanwhile, season the chicken fillet together with your preferred spice blend. Place the bird breast in a greased frying pan and fry the fillets over medium warmness for five-6 minutes.
2. Cut the chicken fillet into cubes after baking. When the broccoli florets are cooked, drain the excess water from the pan.
3. Now heat 2 tbsp olive oil inside the frying pan and add the zucchini spaghetti. Fry the zucchini for 2 minutes after which upload the pesto, broccoli, and chicken. Stir properly and fry for any other 2-3 minutes, till everything within the pan is warm.
4. Divide the contents of the pan among four plates and garnish with pine nuts, Parmesan cheese, cherry tomatoes, and arugula. Enjoy your meal!

NUTRITIONAL VALUES

Serving Size: ¼
Calories: 356
Fats: 19.8
Carbohydrates: 8.9
Proteins: 36.3

Low-carbohydrate detox salad

Cooking time: 25 mins
Total time: 30 mins

INGREDIENTS

- 500 gr raw beets
- 4 carrots or 150 gr raw vegetables carrot julienne
- 100 gr arugula
- 100 gr feta cheese
- 25 ml olive oil
- 15 ml apple cider vinegar

PREPARATION METHOD

1. Take a big slicing board and reduce the ends of the beets away on it. Then peel the beets with a vegetable peeler and reduce a thin slice off the pinnacle and backside if essential. Then rinse the tuber beneath the tap.
2. Now take a huge container and grate all the beets finely above the box. Do the equal with the 4 carrots. Now take four plates and spread the arugula lightly. Add the grated carrot and beets and garnish with the feta cheese.
3. To make the dressing, placed the olive oil and apple cider vinegar in a box and blend nicely. Drizzle the dressing over the detox salad! Enjoy your meal

NUTRITIONAL VALUES

Serving Size: 1 portion
Calories: 168
Fats: 10.3

Carbohydrates: 9.9
Proteins: 6.9

Scrambled eggs with zucchini and shiitake

Cooking time: 10 mins
Total time: 25 mins

INGREDIENTS

- 4 medium eggs
- 1/2 medium zucchini
- 1 small onion
- 40 gr shiitake or chestnut mushrooms
- pepper and salt to taste
- 1 tbsp olive oil
- 1 slice of cheese
- salt and pepper to taste
- optional: clove of garlic

PREPARATION METHOD

1. Grab a massive cutting board and cut the zucchini, onion, and shiitake into small portions. Heat the olive oil in a frying pan over medium warmth. Add the sliced onions and fry for two mins. Add the zucchini and mushrooms and stir fry for 5 minutes extra.
2. Beat the eggs in a bowl and add salt and pepper to flavor. Add the eggs and a slice of cheese to the frying pan and fry with a wood spatula at the same time as stirring. Divide the scrambled eggs over 2 plates and revel in!

NUTRITIONAL VALUES

Serving Size: 1/2 of the scrambled eggs
Calories: 284
Fats: 19.0

Carbohydrates: 8.5
Proteins: 17.5

Low-carbohydrate sausage rolls

Cooking time: 20 mins
Total time: 40 mins

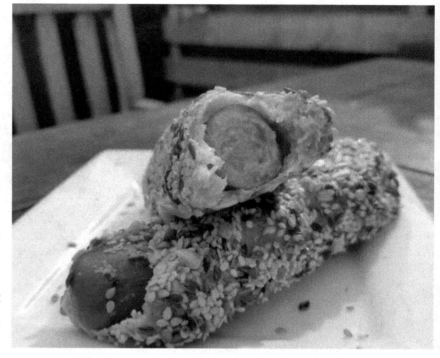

INGREDIENTS

- 4 unox hot dogs
- 120 gr grated mozzarella
- 75 gr almond flour
- 1 tsp xanthan gum
- 2 tbsp cream cheese
- 2 medium eggs
- 4 tbsp seeds & kernels mix (sesame seeds, poppy seeds, linseed)
- 1 - 2 tsp onion powder
- 1 tsp garlic powder

PREPARATION METHOD

1. Place the mozzarella and cream cheese in a microwave-safe bowl and warm within the microwave for 1.5 mins, till the cheese has melted. Mix nicely and set aside.
2. Then preheat the oven to 200 degree. In another bowl, blend the almond flour, 1 egg, and the xanthan gum. Add the cheese mixture to the flour aggregate and knead with wet hands into a lump-loose batter.
3. Shape the dough into four equal-sized balls and vicinity them on a baking tray lined with parchment paper. Carefully roll out each ball with moist palms until it's far approximately 40 cm lengthy.
4. Then wrap each piece of dough tightly around a warm canine and briefly put them on a plate. Then beat the last egg in a bowl with a whisk and spread it over the hot dogs with a brush. Then mix all of the seeds and spices in a bowl and dip the recent puppies inside the spice mixture.
5. Return the new puppies to the baking tray and bake them in the preheated oven till golden brown for 20 mins. Enjoy your meal!

NUTRITIONAL VALUES

Serving Size: 1 hot dog
Calories: 342
Fats: 27.2

Carbohydrates: 4.7
Proteins: 19.5

Low-carbohydrate caprese salad

Cooking time: 20 mins
Total time: 25 mins

INGREDIENTS

- 100 ml balsamic vinegar
- 1 tbsp olive oil
- 2 pieces of chicken fillet (300 gr)
- salt and fresh black pepper
- 200 gr chopped romaine salad
- 150 gr mini mozzarella balls
- 200 gr cherry tomatoes
- 1 avocado, cut into cubes
- handful of basil, finely chopped

PREPARATION METHOD

1. Put the balsamic vinegar in a saucepan and heat over medium warmness. Bring to a light boil and cook dinner for 4-6 minutes, until 50% of the balsamic vinegar has evaporated. Put the closing balsamic vinegar in a container and let it calm down.
2. Heat a tablespoon of olive oil in a skillet over medium warmth. Season the bird breasts with salt and pepper and region in a frying pan. Fry the chook breasts for 4 minutes on every side. Cut the hen breasts into cubes and allow them to calm down.
3. Place the romaine salad in a big bowl and upload the bird, mozzarella, cherry tomatoes, avocado, and basil. Garnish with the balsamic vinegar and divide into 2 quantities.

NUTRITIONAL VALUES

Serving Size: ½
Calories: 475
Fats: 26.0

Carbohydrates: 7.5
Proteins: 50.5

Lettuce wraps filled with turkey fillet and bacon

Cooking time: 10 mins
Total time: 15 mins

INGREDIENTS
Basil Mayonnaise:

- 2 - 3 tbsp mayonnaise
- 6 basil leaves
- optional: 1 small clove of garlic, crushed
- 1 tsp lemon juice

Wraps:

- 1 head of iceberg lettuce
- 6 slices of turkey or chicken fillet
- 4 slices of fried bacon
- 1 small avocado
- 1 Roma tomato
- salt and pepper to taste

PREPARATION METHOD

1. To make the basil mayonnaise, vicinity the mayonnaise, basil, finely overwhelmed garlic, and lemon juice in a small meal processor or blender. Switch at the tool, in brief, to combine the entirety well.
2. Then reduce the avocado and tomato into slices on a large reducing board. Grab the top of iceberg lettuce and tear off the two largest leaves. Put slices of hen or turkey breast on each. Spread a bit of basil mayonnaise on the pinnacle of the fillet slices. On top of this sediment, place another slice of turkey or chicken breast, bacon, tomato slices, and avocado.
3. Season lightly with salt and pepper then fold the lowest of the lettuce wrap up, in the facets, and then roll it close like a burrito. Serve the lettuce wraps cold.

NUTRITIONAL VALUES

Serving Size: 1 wrap
Calories: 300
Fat: 27.5

Carbohydrates: 4.8
Proteins: 12.8

Low-carb cauliflower couscous

Cooking time: 10 mins   **Total time: 25 mins**

INGREDIENTS

- 600 gr cauliflower florets
- 75 gr sundried tomatoes
- 1 - 2 cloves of garlic, finely crushed
- 1 tbsp olive oil
- 150 gr leek, finely chopped
- salt and pepper to taste

- pinch of paprika
- pinch of finely ground cumin
- 1 tbsp lemon juice
- 50 gr walnuts, chopped into pieces
- optional: feta cheese to taste

PREPARATION METHOD

1. Grab a container with water and soak the sun-dried tomatoes in it. Then put the florets of cauliflower in a food processor and grind it granular, similar to real couscous. Add lemon juice to the cauliflower and season with salt, pepper, cumin, and paprika.
2. Grab a medium frying pan and heat a tablespoon of olive oil in it. Add the finely beaten cloves of garlic and the portions of leek and fry for a couple of minutes over medium warmth.
3. Meanwhile, grasp the box with sun-dried tomatoes and permit the water to drain. Then cut the sun-dried tomatoes into small pieces and upload them to the frying pan.
4. Then upload the cauliflower couscous and the walnuts to the pan and fry until executed. Be careful no longer to overcook it, due to the fact then it'll change into a porridge. Divide among four plates and enjoy!

NUTRITIONAL VALUES

Serving Size: ¼

Calories: 230

Fat: 14.5

Carbohydrates: 12.5

Proteins: 5.4

Greek salad of grilled halloumi

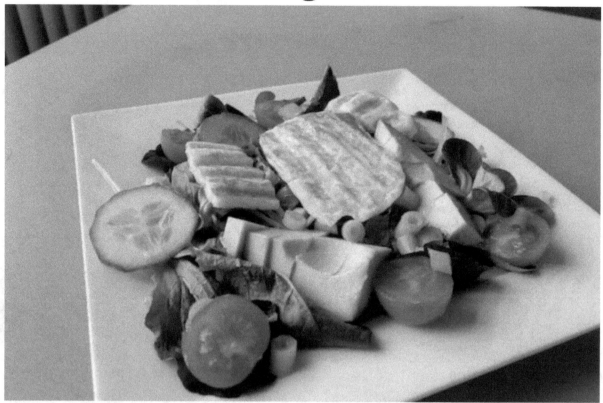

Cooking time: 10 mins   **Total time: 15 mins**

INGREDIENTS

- 225 gr halloumi cheese
- 100 gr salad mix of your choice
- 1 cucumber
- 150 cherry tomatoes
- 4 stalks of spring onion

- 1 avocado
- juice of 1 lemon
- 2 tbsp olive oil
- 1 tbsp balsamic vinegar

PREPARATION METHOD

Grab a large reducing board and cut the spring onion, cherry tomatoes, and cucumber into small pieces on it. Then take the avocado and reduce it in half. Then take away the pit and peel and additionally cut the avocado into small pieces. Put the salad, cucumber, cherry tomatoes, spring onion, avocado in a big bowl and blend the whole lot collectively.

Now take a small bowl and blend in the lemon juice, olive oil, and balsamic vinegar, and set it apart. Then cut the halloumi into frivolously sized slices and location on a hot grill. Grill until the halloumi slices flip brown.

Divide the salad from the bowl over 3 plates and serve with some slices of halloumi and the dressing. Enjoy your meal!

NUTRITIONAL VALUES

Serving Size: 1/3   Carbohydrates: 8.1
Calories: 318   Proteins: 17.6
Fats: 24.1

Vitello tonnato

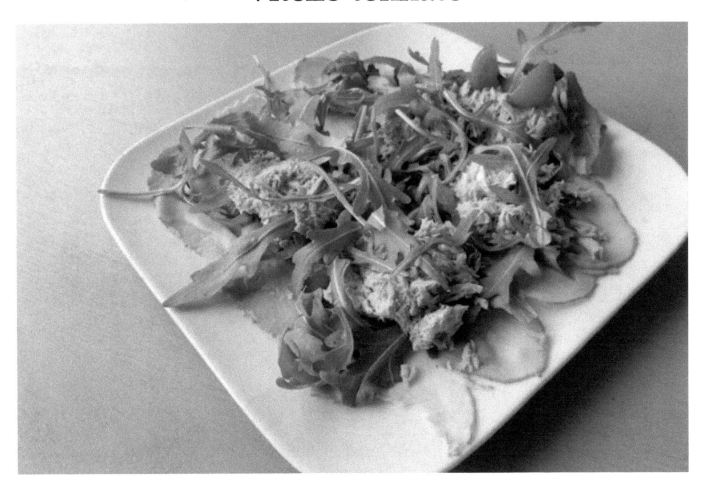

Cooking time: 10 mins   **Total time: 15 mins**

INGREDIENTS

- 185 gr tuna in canned water
- 3 tbsp mayonnaise
- 3 tbsp capers
- lemon juice to taste
- 75 gr arugula
- 200 gr fricandeau
- 50 gr cherry tomatoes

PREPARATION METHOD

1. Divide the fricandeau over two plates. Puree the tuna and mayonnaise with the hand blender. Season with lemon juice, pepper, and salt if desired. Divide the tuna aggregate over the fricandeau and eventually placed the arugula, capers, and tomato over the Vitello tomato.

NUTRITIONAL VALUES

Serving Size: ½

Calories: 364

Fats: 22.6

Carbohydrates: 1.6

Proteins: 36.4

Spicy Indian scrambled eggs with spinach

Cooking time: 15 mins
Total time: 25 mins

INGREDIENTS

- 1 - 2 tsp cumin seeds or cumin powder
- 1 - 2 tsp mustard seeds
- 1 onion, finely chopped
- 25 gr butter
- 1 tbsp olive oil
- 200 gr baby spinach
- 1 tsp garam masala seasoning
- 2 tsp turmeric
- 8 medium eggs
- 4 low- carb wraps
- 3 tsp finely chopped mint
- 6 tbsp yogurt
- salt and black pepper to taste

PREPARATION METHOD

2. Briefly toast the mustard and cumin seeds over low heat in a lightly greased pan. Use a deep frying pan as the seeds can pop up once they get warm. Meanwhile, cut the onion into small portions and upload it to the pan along with a tbsp of butter. Fry the onions until golden brown for approximately five mins. Then add the spinach and fry it till it has gotten smaller and set apart.
3. Then take any other pan and heat the rest of the butter and a little olive oil in it. Add the garam masala and turmeric and cook for 1-2 mins. Meanwhile, beat the eggs in a massive bowl. Add the eggs to the pan and fry whilst stirring.
4. Meanwhile, warmth the wraps inside the oven or in a frying pan. Then take the spinach from the set aside pan and reduce it into small portions and dispose of any extra liquid using a sieve. Add the spinach to the scrambled eggs and prepare dinner for more mins.
5. In-between, reduce the mint into small pieces and upload this to the yogurt in a field. Serve the scrambled eggs with the wrap and yogurt sauce.

NUTRITIONAL VALUES

Serving Size: ¼

Calories: 230

Fats: 15.8

Carbohydrates: 6.1

Proteins: 14.5

Creamy cauliflower risotto

Cooking time: 10 mins
Total time: 15 mins

INGREDIENTS

- 400 gr of cauliflower rice
- 33 gr mascarpone
- 2 tbsp butter
- 25 gr green pesto
- 2 tbsp grated Parmesan cheese
- 1/2 tsp salt
- 1/4 tsp garlic powder
- 1/4 tsp black pepper

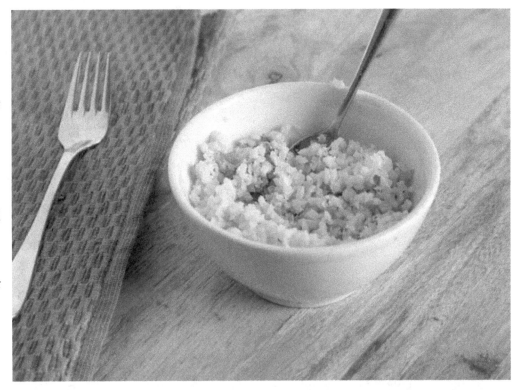

PREPARATION METHOD

1. Heat a tablespoon of butter in a large frying pan or wok pan. Add the cauliflower rice to the pan and fry for 3-4 minutes simultaneously as stirring.
2. Then upload the rest of the butter, mascarpone, and all the herbs and fry for 2 mins while stirring. Finally, add the Parmesan and fry for any other minute.
3. Let cool for 2 mins after adding the green pesto and stir it through the cauliflower risotto. Divide the risotto into portions and enjoy!

NUTRITIONAL VALUES

Serving Size: ½
Calories: 228
Fat: 18.9

Carbohydrates: 10.0
Proteins: 6.8

Adam's low-carb bread

Cooking time: 40 mins   **Total time: 60 min**

INGREDIENTS
- 1 pack of Adam's bread mix white or brown
- 230 ml of lukewarm water

PREPARATION METHOD
1. In a huge bowl, add the bread blend and. Take a tumbler and fill it with 230 ml lukewarm water and add the yeast at the same time as stirring. Then add the yeast and water to the bread mix and knead it by hand for about two mins. Now take a cake tin and positioned the dough in it. Put the cake tin with the dough within the oven for forty-five minutes at 50 degrees so that it may rise properly.
2. When the bread has risen, take it out of the oven and sprinkle the pinnacle with a little water. Bake the bread when it has risen properly for some other 50 minutes within the preheated oven at two hundred degree. Let the bread cool at the counter for half an hour after baking. Cut the bread into thirteen slices and enjoy!

NUTRITIONAL VALUES
Serving Size: 1 slice (35 gr)

Calories: 82

Fats: 3.7

Carbohydrates: 0.2

Proteins: 11.2

Low-carbohydrate chicken meatballs

Cooking time: 15 mins
Total time: 25 mins

INGREDIENTS

Chicken meatballs:

- 450 gr minced chicken
- 1 small zucchini (300 g)
- 2 - 3 stalks of spring onion
- 3 tbsp parsley
- 1 clove of garlic
- 1/2 tsp black pepper
- 1/2 tsp cumin
- 2 tbsp olive oil

Avocado dip:

- 1 avocado
- 1/4 red onion

- 1/2 tomato
- salt and pepper to taste

PREPARATION METHOD

1. Grate the courgette over a big bowl using a hand grater. Then take a clean tea towel and location it on a huge bowl. Spoon the grated zucchini into the tea towel. Lift your clean kitchen towel with the zucchini in it and squeeze out all the moisture. Drain the water inside the bowl and dry it. Then positioned the zucchini in the bowl.

2. On a large reducing board, reduce the spring onion into small portions and upload to the bowl with the zucchini along with the minced chook, parsley, and herbs. Mix the whole thing properly with a fork. Then form about 20 balls of the minced meat mixture with an ice cream scoop or along with your hands.

3. Next, warm two tablespoons of olive oil in a skillet over medium warmness. Add the chook meatballs to the pan and cook dinner for 5 to six mins. Then flip the balls over and bake for another 5 minutes. Then decrease the heat and fry the chook meatballs with the lid on the pan for a few more minutes. It is also viable to bake the chicken meatballs in the oven. Preheat the oven to 205 degree and bake the chicken meatballs for 15-20 mins.

4. You can serve the hen meatballs with a delicious avocado dip. You make this dip using mashing an avocado in a medium bowl. Then reduce the purple onion and tomato into small pieces and add this to the bowl and the lemon juice. Season with salt and pepper, and the dip is finished!

5. Serve the chicken meatballs in keeping with 5 pieces with a little avocado dip and revel in!

NUTRITIONAL VALUES

Serving Size: 5 meatballs

Fat: 25.3

Proteins: 21.3

Calories: 340

Carbohydrates: 5.9

Lettuce wraps with Eastern minced chicken

Cooking time: 20 mins   **Total time: 25 mins**

- 1 tsp rice

INGREDIENTS

- 500 gr natural minced chicken
- 2 tbsp sesame seed oil or wok oil
- 110 gr mushrooms
- 6 g fresh basil
- 2 - 3 tbsp hoisin sauce
- 1 tsp fresh ginger, finely chopped
- 1 tbsp soy sauce
- 2 tsp chopped garlic
- vinegar
- 1 tsp cornstarch
- 1 head of romaine lettuce
- 3 stalks of spring onion

PREPARATION METHOD

1. Cut the mushrooms, spring onion, and basil into small pieces on a massive cutting board. Then warmness the wok oil in a huge frying pan over medium warmness. Add the minced chook to the pan and fry it for about five minutes. Then add the mushrooms and basil to the pan and fry for another 5 mins.
2. Meanwhile, take a small bowl and blend with a whisk the soy sauce, hoisin sauce, ginger, garlic, rice vinegar, and cornstarch. Add the sauce to the minced chicken and permit it to simmer for a couple of minutes. Finally, add the spring onion to the pan.
3. Take the pinnacle of romaine lettuce and punctiliously put off the leaves. Clean the leaves with water and place them on 4 plates. Fill the lettuce leaves with the minced bird and serve with soy sauce. Enjoy your meal!

NUTRITIONAL VALUES

Serving Size: ¼
Calories: 348
Fats: 25.2

Carbohydrates: 6.8
Proteins: 23.5

Low-carb pancakes

Cooking time: 10 mins
Total time: 15 mins

INGREDIENTS

- 4 medium eggs
- 110 ml of water or milk
- 2 - 3 tbsp coconut flour
- 1 tbsp arrowroot or tapioca
- 1 tbsp coconut oil or butter
- 1/2 tsp vanilla aroma
- 1/4 tsp salt
- optional: cinnamon to taste
- optional: erythritol or stevia to taste

PREPARATION METHOD

1. In a medium bowl, combine the coconut flour, arrowroot, and salt. In every other bowl, beat the eggs collectively with the water/milk, coconut oil/butter, and vanilla aroma. Add erythritol and cinnamon to the batter if favored.

2. Add the liquid aggregate to the dry aggregate while stirring and beat until there are no extra lumps. Let the aggregate take a seat for 10 mins to allow the coconut flour to take in moisture.

3. Grease a skillet with butter or oil and warmth over medium heat. Then place 3 tablespoons of the batter within the pan and calmly unfold it. Bake the pancake on one aspect for approximately four minutes. Then flip the pancake with a spatula and prepare dinner the alternative facet for approximately 1 to two mins. Repeat this step till all of the batters are gone, and you have about 8 small or four big pancakes baked.

NUTRITIONAL VALUES

Serving Size: 2 small pancakes
Calories: 88
Fat: 4.8

Carbohydrates: 4.4
Proteins: 6.0

Savory cauliflower pancakes

Cooking time: 15 mins   **Total time: 25 mins**

INGREDIENTS

- 450 g cauliflower rice
- 3 medium eggs
- 50 gr grated cheese
- 2 stalks of spring onion
- salt and pepper to taste

PREPARATION METHOD

1. Cut the spring onion into small portions on a huge slicing board. Then, in a large bowl, integrate the cauliflower rice, eggs, spring onion, cheese, salt, and pepper. After mixing, let the batter relax for 10 mins.
2. In a big frying pan over medium warmness, warmness 2-three tbsp butter. Add a few serving spoons to the frying pan and fry the pancakes (if the pan is huge sufficient several at a time) for 5 mins. Then gently turn them over and bake for another 5 mins. After baking, place the pancakes on a plate and preserve them warm via overlaying the plate with aluminum foil.
3. Repeat step 2 till you run out of batter! Serve the pancakes with a pleasant sauce for breakfast or lunch.

NUTRITIONAL VALUES

Serving Size: 2 pancakes   Fat: 11.3   Proteins: 9.7
Calories: 161   Carbohydrates: 4.7

Lettuce wraps with tuna and avocado dressing

Cooking time: 10 mins
Total time: 20 mins

INGREDIENTS

Lettuce wraps:

- 4 large lettuce leaves (romaine lettuce)
- 1 can of tuna, drained
- 45 gr cherry tomatoes
- 30 gr grated carrot
- 1/2 small red onion

Avocado dressing:

- 125 ml Greek yogurt
- 1/4 small avocado
- 3 tbsp fresh parsley
- optional: 1/2 jalapeño pepper
- 1/2 clove of garlic
- juice of 1/4 lime
- 1/8 tsp salt
- black pepper to taste

PREPARATION METHOD

1. To make the avocado dressing, use a blender or meal processor. Add the yogurt, avocado, parsley, jalapeño, garlic, lime juice, salt, and pepper. Turn on the blender and blend till clean. Add a little water if you think the dressing is just too thick.
2. Then snatch a massive reducing board and reduce the cherry tomatoes and crimson onions into small portions. Then divide the tuna, cherry tomatoes, onion, and carrot over the four lettuce leaves. Drizzle the lettuce leaves with a tablespoon of dressing and serve!

NUTRITIONAL VALUES

Serving Size: 2 lettuce wraps

Calories: 176

Fat: 6.3

Carbohydrates: 6.4

Proteins: 22.3

Low-carbohydrate crepes

Cooking time: 10 mins   **Total time: 25 mins**

INGREDIENTS

- 3 medium eggs
- 85 gr cream cheese (philadelphia)
- 10 gr coconut flour
- 5 gr Steviala Crystal
- 1 tsp cinnamon
- 50 gr strawberries
- optional: sugar-free chocolate or Steviala Frost
- butter or oil

PREPARATION METHOD

1. In a big bowl, mix with a whisk the eggs, coconut flour, Steviala crystal. Then heat the cream cheese in a pan. Then upload the cream cheese to the egg aggregate and mix properly again. Let the batter rest for a couple of minutes.
2. Then heat a tablespoon of butter or oil. Using a soup spoon, add 1/4 of the batter to the pan and flip the pan to distribute the batter.
3. Fry the crepe over a low warmth and turn it over while the bottom is golden brown. Repeat this until the batter is used up. Meanwhile, reduce the strawberries into slices and divide them over the fried pancakes.
4. Garnish the crêpes with melted sugar-unfastened chocolate or Stevia Frost powdered sugar.

NUTRITIONAL VALUES

Serving Size: 1 crepe   Fats: 8.9   Proteins: 5.9

Calories: 114   Carbohydrates: 2.1

Quint's low-carbohydrate bread white multi-seeds

Cooking time: 50 mins
Total time: 50 mins

INGREDIENTS

- 150 gr wheat gluten
- 50 gr soy flour
- 50 gr sesame seeds
- 50 gr sunflower seeds
- 50 g linseed
- 20 gr wheat flour
- 12 gr wheat bran
- 1 sachet of yeast
- 5 g salt
- 270 ml of water

PREPARATION METHOD

1. Preheat the oven to two hundred degree. In a massive bowl, combine the dry elements and add 270ml lukewarm water.
2. Knead the mixture well with your fingers for approximately 2-3 minutes. Form the dough right into a thick roll and location it in a baking tin. Cover with a tea towel and let the bread upward thrust in a heat region for fifty-60 minutes.
3. Bake the bread inside the preheated oven for forty-five mins. Let the bread settle down after baking. Then reduce the bread to 15 slices and revel in!
4. It is likewise feasible to make the bread in the bread maker. Select the wholemeal and 500 g bread weight application in your bread maker. Then placed the mixture's contents together with 270 ml lukewarm water in the machine. Close the lid and start the machine.

NUTRITIONAL VALUES

Serving Size: 1 slice
Calories: 112
Fats: 5.5

Carbohydrates: 3.6
Fiber: 1.9
Proteins: 11.0

Quint's low-carb bread dark pumpkin

Cooking time: 10 mins
Total time: 45 mins

INGREDIENTS

- 140 gr wheat gluten
- 45 gr soy flour
- 45 gr sunflower seeds
- 45 g linseed
- 30 gr pumpkin seeds
- 20 gr wheat flour

- 15 gr sesame seeds
- 12 gr wheat bran
- 7 g yeast (1 sachet)
- 5 g salt
- 3 gr barley malt flour
- 260 ml of water

PREPARATION METHOD

1. Preheat the oven to 200 degree.
2. In a huge bowl, combine the dry components and add 260ml lukewarm water. Knead the combination nicely with your hands for about 2-3 mins. Form the dough right into a thick roll and vicinity it in a baking tin. Cover with a tea towel and let the bread upward thrust in a warm region for 50-60 minutes.
3. Bake the bread in the preheated oven for 45 minutes. Let the bread calm down after baking.
4. You can also bake the bread within the bread maker. Select the wholemeal and 500 g bread weight application in your bread maker. Then position the mix's contents together with 260 ml lukewarm water within the gadget. Close the lid and begin the system.

NUTRITIONAL VALUES

Serving Size: 1 slice (35 gr)
Calories: 109
Fats: 5.2

Carbohydrates: 4.0
Proteins: 10.3

Low-carbohydrate seed crackers

Cooking time: 45 mins
Total time: 75 mins

INGREDIENTS

- 45 gr almond flour
- 45 gr pumpkin seeds
- 50 g linseed
- 50 gr sunflower seeds
- 50 gr sesame seeds
- 1 tbsp psyllium fiber
- 1 tsp salt (or to taste)
- 45 ml coconut oil or olive oil
- 225 ml of boiling water

PREPARATION METHOD

1. Preheat the oven to a hundred and fifty degrees. Then, in a huge bowl, combine all of the dry substances.
2. Boil 230 ml of water in a pan or a kettle. Then add the boiling water and oil to the large bowl with the flour and mix well with a spatula.
3. Place the dough ball among two baking paper sheets and roll out the dough as skinny as viable with a rolling pin.
4. Remove the top parchment paper and location the rolled-out dough on a baking tray.
5. Then area the baking tray at the lowest of the heated oven and bake the low-carb crackers for 45 minutes. While baking, test once to make sure the seeds don't burn.
6. After baking for 45 minutes, flip off the oven and let the low-carb crackers cool inside the oven for 10-15 mins. Then take the baking tray out of the oven and wreck the crackers into the favored length.

NUTRITIONAL VALUES

Serving Size: 1 cracker
Calories: 87
Fats: 7.

6Carbohydrates: 2.5
Fiber: 2.1
Proteins: 2.5

Big Mac salad

Cooking time: 10 mins   **Total time: 20 mins**

INGREDIENTS

Salad :

- 500 gr ground beef
- 400 gr finely chopped iceberg lettuce
- 40 gr chopped onion
- 80 gr grated cheese
- 80 gr gherkin cubes
- 1 tbsp olive oil

- salt and pepper to taste

Big Mac sauce:

- 100 ml of mayonnaise
- 2 tsp mustard
- 2 tbsp finely chopped diced pickles
- 1 tbsp white wine vinegar

- 1 tbsp finely chopped onion
- 1/2 tsp paprika
- 1/2 tsp onion powder
- 1/4 tsp garlic powder

PREPARATION METHOD

1. Heat a tablespoon of olive oil in a frying pan. Add 1/2 of the sliced onions and fry until the onions begin to discolor. Add the floor beef and fry it for five-eight minutes. Season the minced meat with salt and pepper.

2. In the period in-between, we will make the Big Mac sauce. In a big bowl, integrate the mayonnaise, mustard, white wine vinegar, paprika, onion powder, and garlic powder. Then cut the onions and diced pickles greater satisfactory and upload this to the sauce. Let the sauce relax inside the refrigerator to absorb the flavors properly.

3. Drain the moisture from the pan after cooking the minced meat. Then, in a big bowl, combine the iceberg lettuce, sliced onion, diced pickles, grated cheese, and ground red meat.

4. Divide the salad between 4 plates and serve with the Big Mac sauce. Enjoy your meal!

NUTRITIONAL VALUES

Serving Size: 1 portion
Calories: 531
Fats: 43.8

Carbohydrates: 3.7
Proteins: 31.4

Sushi bowl with smoked salmon

Cooking time: 10 mins   **Total time: 15 mins**

INGREDIENTS

Bowl:

- 150 g cauliflower rice
- 1 tbsp olive oil
- 50 gr smoked salmon (cubes)
- 1 - 2 tsp sriracha

- 1/2 cucumber
- 1/2 avocado
- 2 nori sheets
- 1/2 tbsp soy sauce
- 1/2 tsp wasabi, optional

Sauce:

- 2 tbsp mayonnaise

PREPARATION METHOD

1. Heat a tablespoon of olive oil in a big frying pan. Add the cauliflower rice to the pan and cook for two-three minutes. Season the cauliflower rice with soy sauce, salt, and pepper
2. Then reduce the avocado and smoked salmon into cubes. You can prepare the cucumber in two ways. You can cut the cucumber into cubes or form it into strings with the usage of a spiral cutter. Finally, cut the nori sheets into small squares.
3. Place all elements in a bowl and serve with the wasabi and the sriracha mayo. The sriracha mayo is made by mixing 2 tbsp mayonnaise with a 1-2 tsp sriracha. Enjoy your meal!

NUTRITIONAL VALUES

Serving Size: 1 bowl   Fats: 39.9   Proteins: 16.6

Calories: 478   Carbohydrates: 9.3

Low-carbohydrate chaffle waffles

Cooking time: 10 mins
Total time: 15 mins

INGREDIENTS

- 60 gr grated mozzarella
- 1 tbsp almond flour
- 1 egg (M or L)
- butter or coconut oil for greasing
- 20 gr grated cheese (mozzarella or Gouda)

PREPARATION METHOD

1. Heat the waffle iron and grease it with a touch of butter or coconut oil.
2. Meanwhile, in a bowl, blend the 60 g grated mozzarella, almond flour, and the egg.
3. Sprinkle a bit little bit of grated cheese (mozzarella or Gouda) at the waffle iron and then upload the batter. Then sprinkle a few grated slices of cheese on top of the wafer and close the waffle iron. Bake the cheese wafer for approx. 6-eight mins within the waffle iron.

NUTRITIONAL VALUES

Serving Size: 1 large wafer   Fats: 25.2   Proteins: 24.0
Calories: 336   Carbohydrates: 2.5

Egg wrap with salmon and spinach

Cooking time: 10 mins
Total time: 15 mins

INGREDIENTS

- 3 medium eggs
- dash of almond milk
- 100 g baby spinach
- 2 tbsp olive oil
- salt and pepper to taste
- 25 gr cream cheese
- 20 gr arugula
- 50 gr smoked salmon
- 4 cherry tomatoes
- 1/4 tsp salt
- optional: handful of pine nuts

PREPARATION METHOD

1. Cut the child spinach into small pieces on a huge board. Then warmness a tablespoon of olive oil in a medium frying pan and fry the child spinach for approx. 2 mins. In a large bowl with a whisk, combine the eggs, almond milk, and salt. After cooking the spinach, drain the extra from the pan and add the spinach to the bowl and mix properly with the eggs.
2. Fry the spinach omelet in the same frying pan over a low warmness within 5-10 mins. If feasible, turn the omelet carefully with a spatula halfway via cooking.
3. Let the omelet cool for at least half-hour, after which cut the cherry tomatoes into small slices. When the omelet has cooled, unfold the cream cheese over the omelet and coat with the arugula, smoked salmon, cherry tomatoes, and pine nuts. Roll the omelet tightly, reduce in 1/2 and enjoy!

NUTRITIONAL VALUES

Serving Size: 1/2 egg wrap

Calories: 236

Fat: 17.5

Carbohydrates: 1.9

Proteins: 16.5

Almond flour pancakes

Cooking time: 30 mins
Total time: 35 mins

INGREDIENTS

- 2 large eggs
- 125 ml almond milk
- 2 tbsp coconut oil or olive oil
- 1 tsp vanilla aroma
- 100 gr almond flour
- 2 tbsp erythritol or Steviala Kristal to taste
- 1 tsp baking powder
- pinch of salt

PREPARATION METHOD

1. Add the eggs, almond milk, vanilla flavoring, and coconut oil to a big blender. Run the blender for approximately 30 seconds to mix everything collectively. Then upload the almond flour, baking powder, erythritol, and salt to the blender and blend for some other 30 seconds. After blending, allow the batter relaxation for five minutes.

2. Then take a massive frying pan and heat a tablespoon of butter or oil in it. Spoon three tablespoons of the batter into the pan and fry the pancake until bubbles form on the floor of the pancake, about 2-three minutes. Then flip the pancake and cook for any other 2-3 minutes. Repeat this step till you've got baked 10 pancakes. Enjoy your meal!

NUTRITIONAL VALUES

Serving Size: 2 pancakes
Calories: 174

Fat: 15.6
Carbohydrates: 1.8

Proteins: 6.7

Low-carb pumpkin soup

Cooking time: 10 mins
Total time: 20 mins

INGREDIENTS

- 400 gr pumpkin (cubes)
- 2 tomatoes
- 1 onion
- 1 leek
- 1 clove of garlic, finely crushed
- 100 ml of cooking cream
- 700 ml of water
- 1 vegetable stock cube
- 125 gr sour cream
- parsley to taste
- salt and pepper to taste.
- 1 tbsp olive oil or butter

PREPARATION METHOD

1. Dice the pumpkin, onion, leek, and tomatoes on a massive cutting board. Grab a big stockpot and heat a tablespoon of butter or olive oil in it. Add the onions and garlic to the pan and fry for 1-2 mins, till the onion starts to discolor. Then upload the relaxation of the veggies and fry for three mins whilst stirring.
2. Add the water to the pan and fall apart the stock dice over the pan. Bring the contents of the pan to a boil and cook dinner for 20 mins over a low warmness.
3. After 20 minutes of cooking, remove the pan from the heat and use a hand blender to mash the contents of the pan into a smooth soup. Then add the cooking cream and cook it for two mins. Taste the soup and season with a touch of salt and pepper is essential.
4. Divide the soup amongst 4 bowls, garnish with parsley and spoon a tbsp sour cream into every bowl. Enjoy your meal!

NUTRITIONAL VALUES

Serving Size: 1 bowl
Calories: 142
Fats: 12.3
Carbohydrates: 6.8
Proteins: 2.9

Thai Beef Salad

Total time: 75 mins

Cooking time: 10 mins

INGREDIENTS

Marinade

- 2 tsp grated ginger
- 2 cloves of garlic
- 1/2 tsp chopped lemon grass (Go-Tan)
- 1/2 shallot, finely chopped
- 2 tbsp fish sauce
- optional: 1 tsp honey

Salad

- 300 gr steak
- 200 gr romaine lettuce
- 1 shallot
- 2 stalks of spring onion

- handful of fresh mint
- 1 red or green peppers
- 1 cucumber
- 3 tbsp peanuts or cashews
- 30 gr butter for baking or roasting

Dressing

- 2 tbsp soy sauce
- 1 tbsp fish sauce
- 2 tbsp lime juice
- 1 tsp grated ginger
- optional: 1 tsp honey

PREPARATION METHOD

1. To make the marinade, upload the ginger, garlic, lemongrass, shallot, and fish sauce to a blender and flip it on till nicely mixed. Then grasp a metal container and put the steak in it. Pour the marinade over the steak and close the box. Put the container within the fridge and allow the marinade to soak for a minimum of an hour.
2. Then reduce the romaine lettuce, spring onion, cucumber, bell pepper, mint, shallot, and peanuts into small portions on a big slicing board and divide this over bowls.
3. Remove the marinated steak from the refrigerator and permit it relaxation at room temperature for 15 minutes. Then heat the butter in a frying pan and while the froth disappears, add the steak to the pan. Fry the steak for two-three minutes per side or rare, medium, or properly done as desired.
4. Meanwhile, make the dressing by using blending nicely the soy sauce, fish sauce, lime juice, and ginger in a small bowl. Cut the fried steak into strips and divide this along with the dressing over the 2 bowls. Enjoy your meal!
5.

NUTRITIONAL VALUES

Serving Size: 1 small bowl
Calories: 348
Fat: 15.4
Carbohydrates: 10.4
Proteins: 41.5

Low-carbohydrate frikandel salad

Cooking time: 10 mins
Total time: 15 mins

INGREDIENTS
Frikandel special:
- 2 Mora oven frikandellen
- 10 gr Heinz tomato ketchup 0% sugar
- 10 gr mayonnaise or French fries sauce
- 15 g onion chips

Salad:
- 75 gr arugula salad mix
- 1/4 cucumber
- 4 cherry tomatoes
- 35 gr mini mozzarella balls
- 2 tsp balsamic vinegar

PREPARATION METHOD
1. Heat the convection oven to 220 degree. Line a baking tray with parchment paper and area the frozen frikandels on the baking tray. Put the frikandels in the oven and bake them within 8-10 mins. You also can put together the frikandels within the air fryer. Then bake the frikandels at 2 hundred degree for six-eight minutes.
2. Meanwhile, make the salad using reducing the cucumber and cherry tomatoes into small cubes. Then upload the arugula salad mix, the chopped components, the mini mozzarella balls, and the balsamic vinegar to a massive bowl and mix nicely. Serve the salad on a huge plate or a small bowl.
3. After baking, do away with the frikandels from the oven or air fryer and cut the frikandels in half lengthwise; however, do now not cut them. Pipe a bit of mayonnaise and sugar-free ketchup into the hole of the frikandelles and garnish with chopped onions. Serve the frikandels with the salad. Enjoy your meal!

NUTRITIONAL VALUES
Serving Size: 1 portion

Calories: 495

Fats: 36.7

Carbohydrates: 13.8

Proteins: 27.6

Chocolate pancakes

Cooking time: 15 mins
Total time: 30 mins

INGREDIENTS

- 3 large eggs
- 125 ml of whole milk
- 1 tsp vanilla aroma
- 150 gr almond flour
- 4 tbsp erythritol
- 2 tbsp melted butter
- 2 tbsp cocoa powder
- 1 tsp baking powder
- butter for frying
- optional: Steviala Frost

PREPARATION METHOD

1. In a medium bowl, integrate the eggs, vanilla taste, milk, erythritol, and melted butter. Using a sieve, add the almond flour to the bowl and stir it through the opposite components with a whisk till all the massive lumps are long gone. Then upload the cocoa powder and baking powder and mix nicely.
2. Next, warm a little butter in a big frying pan and position 3 tablespoons of the batter inside the pan. Fry the pancake for two minutes per facet over a low to medium warmth. Repeat this until you have got baked 12 small pancakes or 6 large pancakes. Serve the pancakes with whipped cream, Steviala frost, and raspberries if preferred. Enjoy your meal!

NUTRITIONAL VALUES

Serving Size: 2 pancakes (2/12)
Calories: 240
Fats: 20.4

Carbohydrates: 3.1
Fiber: 2.1
Proteins: 9.4

Carpaccio salad

Cooking time: 10 mins
Total time: 10 mins

INGREDIENTS

- 240 gr carpaccio (2 packs)
- 150 gr arugula salad mix
- 200 gr cherry tomatoes
- 100 gr radish
- 1 cucumber
- 20 gr capers
- 40 gr pine nuts
- 40 gr Parmesan cheese
- 4 tbsp pesto
- 1 tsp lemon juice

PREPARATION METHOD

1. Cut the cherry tomatoes in half, the cucumber in slices, and the radishes in thin slices. Then take the carpaccio and cut the slices into smaller pieces. Then roast the pine nuts for approx—1 minutes in a frying pan without oil.
2. Divide the arugula salad mix and carpaccio over four plates and drizzle with the carpaccio packaging's furnished dressing. Add the tomatoes, cucumber, radishes, and capers to lettuce plates, and finally garnish the salad with Parmesan cheese, green pesto, and lemon juice. Enjoy your meal!

NUTRITIONAL VALUES

Serving Size: 1/4 of the salad
Calories: 280
Fat: 18.5
Carbohydrates: 7.2
Fiber: 2.5
Proteins: 19.6

Low-carbohydrate tomato soup

Cooking time: 25 mins
Total time: 30 mins
INGREDIENTS

- 6 large roma or vine tomatoes (500 gr)
- 1 tbsp olive oil
- 1 onion
- 1 clove of garlic
- 1 stalk of celery
- 1 winter carrot
- 1 tbsp Italian herbs
- 1 tbsp tomato paste
- 1 vegetable stock cube
- 1 liter of water
- 250 gr ground beef
- salt and pepper to taste
- optional: dash of cooking cream

Preparation method

1. Cut the onion, carrot, and celery into small pieces and weigh down the garlic with a garlic press. Then cast off the crown from the tomatoes and reduce a go at the tomatoes' bottom with a small knife. Dip the tomatoes in boiling water for 10 seconds and put them in cold water straight away. Carefully peel the skins from the tomatoes with the knife. Then reduce the skinned tomatoes into small portions.

2. Heat a tablespoon of olive oil in a stockpot. Add the sliced onion and pressed garlic to the pan and fry until the onion starts to discolor. Then add the portions of celery, carrot, and tomato puree to the pan and fry for 2-3 minutes. Then add the tomato pieces to the pan and the Italian herbs and simmer for five mins over a low warmness.

3. Then add 1 liter of water at the side of an inventory cube to the pan and produce it to the boil. Simmer the contents of the pan over low warmth for 20 minutes. After boiling, eliminate the pan from the heat and use a hand blender to mash the pan's contents into a smooth soup.

4. After mashing, put the pan returned on the fire. Then form small balls from the minced meat and upload them to the soup. Boil the balls within the soup for at least five minutes. After cooking, season the soup with salt and pepper. Divide the tomato soup into 5-6 portions and serve with clean parsley and a dash of cooking cream if favored. Enjoy your meal!

NUTRITIONAL VALUES

Serving Size: 1 bowl (1/6)
Calories: 158
Fats: 10.6

Carbohydrates: 5.0
Fiber: 1.6
Proteins: 8.4

Low-carbohydrate nut bread

Cooking time: 60 mins
Total time: 70 mins

INGREDIENTS

- 100 gr walnuts
- 100 gr sunflower seeds
- 100 gr linseed
- 50 gr sesame seeds
- 50 gr pumpkin seeds
- 50 gr almonds
- 50 gr almond flour
- 4 eggs
- 50 ml olive oil or coconut oil
- 1 teaspoon salt (5 grams)

PREPARATION METHOD

1. Preheat the convection oven to 160 degrees. In a large bowl, combine the nuts, seeds, salt and
2. Preheat the convection oven to 160 ranges. In a big bowl, combine the nuts, seeds, salt, and almond flour. Then upload the eggs and olive oil and mix the bowl's contents nicely with a whisk.
3. Cover a loaf tin with baking paper and pour it into the tin. Divide the batter flippantly over the mold with a spoon and slide the mildew with the batter into the oven.
4. Bake the nut bread inside the preheated oven for 60 minutes. Let the bread settle down after baking. Cut the bread into 20 slices of 35 grams after cooling.

NUTRITIONAL VALUES

Serving Size: 1 slice (35 gr)
Calories: 183
Fats: 16.1

Carbohydrates: 1.6
Fiber: 2.9
Proteins: 6.7

Cucumber rolls with chicken

Cooking time: 10 mins
Total time: 10 mins

INGREDIENTS

- 1 cucumber, chilled
- 40 gr green pesto
- 1 scoop of mozzarella
- 80 gr chicken fillet (slices)
- 1/4 red bell pepper
- handful of arugula
- handful of pine nuts

PREPARATION METHOD

1. Wash the cucumber and reduce the ends off. Then take a cheese slicer and use it to slice the cucumber into long slices. Place the long slices on a paper towel to permit the excess moisture to drain out. Meanwhile, cut the red pepper and bird fillet into small portions and the mozzarella into thin slices.

2. Pat every slice of cucumber dry and then spread the slices with a little green pesto. Cover the slices with chook breast, mozzarella, strips

of bell pepper, arugula, and pine nuts. Roll up the slices tightly and relaxed them with a skewer. Enjoy your meal!

NUTRITIONAL VALUES

Serving Size: 1 portion (5 rolls)
Calories: 315
Fats: 22.6
Carbohydrates: 6.1
Fiber: 0.8
Proteins: 20.7

Low-carbohydrate quesadilla

Cooking time: 10 mins
Total time: 20 mins

INGREDIENTS

- 150 gr chicken cubes
- 2 tbsp olive oil
- 1/2 tbsp taco seasoning
- 1/4 red bell pepper
- 1/2 onion
- 2 low- carb wraps from Atkins
- 50 gr grated cheddar or Mexican cheese
- optional: sour cream or salsa

PREPARATION METHOD

1. Heat a tablespoon of olive oil in a big frying pan. Add the chicken cubes to the pan and fry for approximately 5 minutes simultaneously as stirring. Meanwhile, reduce the onion and bell pepper into small portions.

2. When the hen is cooked, upload the chopped onion, bell pepper, and taco seasoning to the pan and fry for three to 5 mins. Then scoop the pan's contents right into a bowl and clean the pan.

3. Now take the wraps and rub one aspect of every wrap with a bit of olive oil. Place a wrap oil-aspect down on a board and sprinkle half of the grated cheese on the wrap. Then spoon the

chicken filling on the wrap and sprinkle the rest of the cheese on top—finally, location the opposite tortilla oil-side up on top of the filled wrap.

4. Heat the skillet over medium heat and upload the filled quesadilla to the pan. Put the lid at the pan and bake the quesadilla for two-4 mins. Then gently turn the quesadilla with a spatula or cheese slicer and bake for some other 2 mins.

5. Remove the quesadilla from the pan after baking and reduce it into four portions. Divide the 4 portions over 2 plates and serve with salsa or bitter cream if favored. Enjoy your meal!

NUTRITIONAL VALUES

Serving Size: 1/2 quesadilla
Calories: 413
Fats: 23.6
Carbohydrates: 8.0
Fiber: 11.7
Proteins: 33.6

Omelette with bacon and tomato

Cooking time: 5 mins
Total time: 10 mins

INGREDIENTS

- 2 eggs
- splash of milk
- 1 tbsp butter or olive oil
- 20 gr grated cheese
- 3 slices of bacon
- 30 gr cherry tomatoes
- 1/2 tbsp chives
- salt and pepper to taste

PREPARATION METHOD

1. Cut the cherry tomatoes into small pieces and the chives on a large cutting board. Beat the eggs with the milk in a bowl and season with salt and pepper. Then, warm a frying pan over medium warmness and fry the bacon until crispy. Remove the bacon from the pan after cooking and region it on a paper towel.

2. Return the pan to heat and upload a tbsp olive oil. When the oil is warm, pour the beaten eggs into the pan. Move the pan to and fro so that the complete backside is blanketed with egg—Fry the omelet for two minutes over a low warmness.

3. Sprinkle the omelet with grated cheese and cook dinner for some other 2 mins with the pan's lid. Then dispose of the lid from the pan and divide the fried bacon, sliced tomatoes, and chives over the omelet. Fold the omelet in half with a spatula and serve on a warm plate. Enjoy your meal!

NUTRITIONAL VALUES

Serving Size: 1 omelet
Calories: 410
Fat: 33.4
Carbohydrates: 3.5
Proteins: 23.7

APPETIZER

Low-carbohydrate sajoer beans

Cooking time: 15 mins
Total time: 25 mins

INGREDIENTS

- 500 gr green beans
- 1 onion
- 1 clove of garlic
- 2 cm fresh ginger
- 1 tsp laos herbs
- 2 to 3 tsp sambal oelek
- 1 tbsp olive oil
- 1 tsp soy sauce
- 200 ml coconut milk
- 1/2 vegetable stock cube

PREPARATION METHOD

1. Clean the green beans and cut the ends of the beans off. Add the green beans to a pan of boiling water and pre-prepare dinner for five-6 mins.
2. Meanwhile, add the onion, garlic, ginger, galangal, and sambal to a blender and mix right into a first-rate paste. After cooking, placed the beans in a colander and ensure that each extra liquid has tired.
3. Heat a tablespoon of olive oil in a frying pan and upload the spice paste to the pan. Then add the green beans and fry for 2-three mins while stirring. Then upload the coconut milk and soy sauce and collapse the stock dice over the pan.
4. Stew the green beans over a low warmth within 5-8 mins. Divide the beans among four plates and serve with cauliflower rice and rendang if desired.

NUTRITIONAL VALUES

Serving Size: 1 portion (1/3)
Calories: 191

Fats: 14.8
Carbohydrates: 5.8

Fiber: 7.5
Proteins: 5.3

Fresh cucumber salad

Cooking time: 10 mins   **Total time: 10 mins**

INGREDIENTS

- 2 cucumbers
- 1/2 red onion
- 125 gr Greek yogurt

- 1 tbsp white wine vinegar
- 1 tbsp fresh dill, finely chopped

- 1/4 tsp salt
- 1/4 tsp garlic powder

PREPARATION METHOD.

1. Clean the cucumber and reduce it into thin slices with a cheese slicer or a sharp knife. Then cut the crimson onion into earrings and upload it to a large bowl along with the cucumber.
2. In every other bowl, mix the Greek yogurt with the white wine vinegar, sliced dill, salt, and garlic powder. Add the dressing to the cucumber salad and mix well.
3. Divide the cucumber salad over 4 plates and garnish with more dill or red onion if desired. Enjoy your meal!

NUTRITIONAL VALUES

Serving Size: 1 portion (1/4   Fats: 3.8   Proteins: 2.7

Calories: 67   Carbohydrates: 4.4

Cauliflower salad with cheese

Cooking time: 15 mins
Total time: 25 mins

INGREDIENTS

cauliflowers lade

- 400 gr cauliflower
- 1 red pepper
- 200 gr sliced red cabbage (fresh)
- 2 stalks of celery
- 2 stalks of spring onion
- 100 gr cheese cubes or feta

Dressing

- 4 tbsp olive oil
- lemon juice from 1/2 lemon
- handful of basil finely chopped

PREPARATION METHOD

1. Cut the cauliflower into florets and cook the florets al dente for approximately five-eight mins. It is likewise viable to roast the cauliflower. To do that, drizzle the cauliflower with olive oil and bake the florets at two hundred degrees for 15-20 mins.
2. Meanwhile, reduce the bell pepper, celery, and spring onion into small portions. Add this to a bowl and blend nicely. Nowcast off the cauliflower from the oven or pan and allow the excess moisture to drain. Let the cauliflower cool down for some time, and then season with salt and pepper.
3. Add the cold cauliflower to the bowl with the opposite vegetables and blend properly again. Now make the dressing by blending the olive oil, lemon juice, and basil in a small bowl.
4. Divide the salad among three plates. Finally, reduce the cheese cubes into even smaller cubes and serve the salad with the dressing and cheese cubes. Enjoy your meal!

NUTRITIONAL VALUES

Serving size: 1/3 of the total
Calories: 268

Fats: 19.8
Carbohydrates: 7.8

Fiber: 5.8
Proteins: 12.1

Fresh green salad

Cooking time: 10 mins
Total time: 10 mins

INGREDIENTS

Salad:

- 150 gr salad mix
- 1 cucumber
- 125 gr cherry tomatoes
- 1/2 red onion
- 100 gr radishes
- handful of pine nuts
- handful of sunflower seeds

Dressing:

- 35 ml olive oil
- 1 tbsp lemon juice
- 1/2 tbsp vinegar
- 1 tsp mustard
- 1/2 tsp garlic powder
- salt and pepper to taste

PREPARATION METHOD

1. Quarter the cucumber and cherry tomatoes. Then take the radishes and smooth them. Cut the radishes into thin slices and set them apart. Then peel the onion and cut it into thin rings.
2. Mix all of the French dressing substances in a bowl with a whisk.
3. Divide the lettuce blend over 4 plates and garnish the plates with the pieces of cucumber, tomato, radish, onion, pine nuts, and sunflower seeds. Serve the salad with the French dressing. Enjoy your meal!

NUTRITIONAL VALUES

Serving Size: 1/4 of the salad
Calories: 148

Fats: 12.4
Carbohydrates: 4.3

Proteins: 3.6

Rutabaga fries

Cooking time: 30 mins
Total time: 35 mins

INGREDIENTS

- 400 gr turnips
- 2 tbsp olive oil
- 1 tsp cayenne pepper
- 1 tsp paprika powder
- 1/2 tsp garlic powder
- salt and pepper to taste
- optional: fries herbs

PREPARATION METHOD

1. Peel the kohlrabi cut them into small fries, or use ready-made kohlrabi fries. Fill a pan with salted water and bring it to a boil. Add the turnip fries to the pan and cook for three-5 mins.
2. After cooking, pour the contents of the pan right into a colander and allow the excess liquid to drain nicely. Then pat the swede fries dry with a paper towel. Place the fries on a baking tray coated with parchment paper and add the olive oil and herbs. Mix the whole lot properly with your palms so that the herbs and oil are frivolously disbursed.
3. For preparation in the oven: preheat the oven to two hundred ranges. Place the baking tray within the oven and bake the turnip fries for 25-half-hour within the preheated oven.
4. For education inside the air fryer: preheat the air fryer at one hundred eighty degree. Put the turnip fries inside the basket and bake for 12 mins at a hundred and eighty degree. Then increase the temperature to 2 hundred ranges and bake for another 5 minutes for a crispy layer. Serve the fries with sugar-loose ketchup and mayonnaise. Enjoy your meal!

NUTRITIONAL VALUES

Serving size: 1/2 of the total
Calories: 110

Fat: 9.2
Carbohydrates: 4.0

Proteins: 2.0

Green asparagus with Parma ham

Cooking time: 10 mins
Total time: 15 mins

INGREDIENTS

- 400 gr green asparagus
- 100 gr Prosciutto di Parma (Parma ham)
- 40 g grated parmesan cheese
- 1 - 2 tbsp olive oil
- salt and pepper to taste
- lemon juice to taste (optional)

PREPARATION METHOD

1. Preheat the convection oven to two hundred degree and line a baking tray with a parchment paper sheet. Clean the asparagus with touch water and reduce away the difficult ends.
2. Then cut the slices of Parma ham in half. Sprinkle the slices of Parma ham with a touch of grated parmesan cheese. Then wrap a slice of Parma ham with parmesan cheese tightly around one asparagus and repeat until all of the asparagus has a slice of ham.
3. Then region the asparagus at the baking tray and sprinkle with the last grated parmesan cheese, and drizzle with the olive oil. Finally, season the asparagus with a little salt and pepper.
4. Bake the asparagus inside the preheated oven for eight-10 minutes. The asparagus is finished if they bend slightly while picked up. After frying, divide asparagus into four quantities and serve with a balsamic sauce if favored. Enjoy your meal!

NUTRITIONAL VALUES

Serving size: 1/4 of the total
Calories: 161

Fat: 11.3
Carbohydrates: 3.3

Fiber: 1.5
Proteins: 11.0

Casserole with green beans

Cooking time: 20 mins
Total time: 35 mins

INGREDIENTS

- 600 gr green beans
- 250 gr mushrooms
- 125 gr bacon strips
- 2 shallots, finely chopped
- 250 ml of cooking cream
- 50 gr cream cheese
- 30 g grated parmesan cheese
- salt and pepper to taste
- optional: cayenne pepper to taste

PREPARATION METHOD

1. Preheat the oven to 180 degree. Then reduce the mushrooms into slices and the onion into small cubes. Then take a massive frying pan and fry the bacon in it until tender and crispy. After frying, put the bacon in a bowl and blot away the excess fats.

2. Fry the chopped onion and mushrooms in the equal frying pan over medium warmth within approx. Three minutes. Then add the cooking cream, cream cheese, and herbs to the pan. Bring this to the boil while stirring and preparing dinner for about four minutes, till the sauce starts to thicken. Then lower the warmth and simmer for any other 6-eight minutes to thicken the sauce further.

3. Meanwhile, grab a massive pan and fill it with water. Add the green beans and a pinch of salt to the pan and cook dinner the green beans for about 8-10 minutes until al dente. After cooking, drain the green beans properly and pat dry with a paper towel if necessary.

4. Then add the cooked green beans to the pan with the mushroom sauce and blend well with a spatula. Spoon the pan's contents into an oven dish and bake for 15 mins in the preheated oven.

5. After 15 mins, dispose of the dish from the oven and sprinkle with the fried bacon and parmesan cheese. Then go back the casserole to the oven and bake for another 5 minutes. Divide into four portions after baking. Enjoy your meal!

NUTRITIONAL VALUES

Serving Size: 1/4 of the dish
Calories: 260

Fats: 18.1
Carbohydrates: 11.8

Fiber: 7.2
Proteins: 10.0

Sugar snaps from the oven

Cooking time: 10 mins   **Total time: 15 mins**

INGREDIENTS

- 225 gr sugar snaps
- 40 gr grated Parmesan cheese
- 15 ml of olive oil
- 15 g shallots, cut into pieces
- 1 tsp fresh thyme, chopped into pieces
- salt and pepper to taste

PREPARATION METHOD.

1. Preheat the oven to 225 ranges. Then take the sparkling sugar snaps and get rid of the ends and any threads. Spread the sugar snaps on a baking tray covered with parchment paper and brush the sugar snaps with olive oil. Then sprinkle the Parmesan cheese shallots, thyme, and sea salt over the sugar snaps.
2. Bake the sugar snaps within the preheated oven for 6-10 minutes. Divide into 4 equal portions and serve!

NUTRITIONAL VALUES

Serving Size: ¼   Fats: 6.2   Proteins: 5.0

Calories: 93   Carbohydrates: 3.6

cauliflower Purée

Cooking time: 10 mins   **Total time: 18 mins**

INGREDIENTS

- 1 medium cauliflower
- 2 - 3 tsp finely ground garlic
- 4 tbsp butter
- 1/2 tsp salt
- 1/2 tsp pepper
- olive oil to taste

PREPARATION METHOD

1. Take the cauliflower and cut away all brown and black spots. Then cast off the cauliflower leaves and reduce the cauliflower into small pieces.
2. Boil or steam the cauliflower in a saucepan with water for approximately 10-15 minutes. After cooking, pour away the excess water using a lid or colander. Then put the cauliflower, butter, garlic, and other herbs in a large bowl and blend until easy with a hand blender. If you do not have a stick blender, you could additionally mix substances in a blender or meal processor. Divide into 4 quantities and serve! Garnish with a little olive oil and further clean black pepper if favored.

NUTRITIONAL VALUES

Serving Size: ¼   Fats: 12.4   Proteins: 2.9

Calories: 142   Carbohydrates: 8.0

Fried Brussels sprouts with pecans

Cooking time: 10 mins   **Total time: 20 mins**

INGREDIENTS

- 350 gr Brussels sprouts
- 40 gr pecans
- 20 gr dried dates
- 2 tbsp olive oil
- 1 tsp apple cider vinegar
- 1 tsp mustard
- 1 tbsp butter

PREPARATION METHOD

1. Clean the Brussels sprouts and blanch them in boiling water for 3 minutes. Meanwhile, cut the pecans in half and, in short, toast them in a dry frying pan.
2. In a small bowl, combine the olive oil, apple cider vinegar, mustard, salt, and pepper. Drain the Brussels sprouts and rinse with cold water. Then warmness a tablespoon of butter in a frying pan and fry the Brussels sprouts for three to four minutes until al dente.
3. Meanwhile, reduce the dates into small portions. Cut the Brussels sprouts in half after baking. In a huge bowl, blend the Brussels sprouts with the nuts and fruits and warm the whole thing up a bit longer. Pour the dressing over the Brussels sprouts and enjoy!

NUTRITIONAL VALUES

Serving Size: 1/3   Fats: 18.6   Proteins: 5.8

Calories: 239   Carbohydrates: 8.6

Low-carb fries

Cooking time: 20 mins   **Total time: 40 mins**

INGREDIENTS

- 1/2 celeriac
- 1 tbsp olive oil
- 1 tsp paprika powder
- 1/2 tsp salt
- 1/4 tsp black pepper

PREPARATION METHOD

1. Preheat an oven to 205 ranges. Take the celeriac and put off the skin and cut the flesh into very thin fries. Put the fries in a bowl and blend with the herbs and olive oil.
2. Then take a baking tray coated with parchment paper and spread the fries frivolously at the baking tray. Bake the fries for 20 to 40 mins inside the preheated oven (relies upon the thickness of the fries), shaking on occasion while baking. Serve with a sauce and experience!

NUTRITIONAL VALUES

Serving Size: 1/3   Fats: 4.0   Proteins: 1.0

Calories: 47   Carbohydrates: 3.0

Low-carbohydrate coleslaw

Cooking time: 10 mins   **Total time: 15 mins**

INGREDIENTS

- 200 gr white cabbage, finely chopped
- 150 gr red cabbage, finely chopped
- 100 gr grated carrot
- 10 radishes
- 1 stalk of spring onion
- 150 gr of sour cream
- 65 ml mayonnaise
- 1 tbsp lemon juice
- 1/8 tsp onion powder
- 1/4 tsp black pepper

PREPARATION METHOD

1. On a large cutting board, cut the radishes into strips and the spring onion into small pieces. Then, in a big bowl, integrate the white cabbage, pink cabbage, grated carrot, spring onion, and radishes.
2. Then snatch every other bowl and blend within the mayonnaise, sour cream, and herbs. Then stir the dressing into the coleslaw. Divide into 6 quantities and serve with lemon juice.

NUTRITIONAL VALUES

Serving Size: 1/6   Fat: 11.8   Proteins: 2.2
Calories: 129   Carbohydrates: 4.5

Cauliflower Rice

Cooking time: 15 mins
Total time: 25 mins

INGREDIENTS

- 1 medium cauliflower
- food processor or grater

PREPARATION METHOD

1. Preheat the oven to 200 degree. Take the cauliflower and cut away all brown and black spots. Then dispose of the leaves from the cauliflower. Cut the cauliflower in half and put off the stump. Cut what's left of the cauliflower into florets of the same length.
2. Then placed the florets in the meal processor and pulverized them into rice (not completely floor). If you do not have a meal processor, you may additionally use a grater; this takes a little longer.
3. Get a baking tray covered with parchment paper. Place the cauliflower rice in a single layer on the baking sheet. Bake the rice inside the preheated oven for 12 minutes. Flip the rice as a minimum as soon as at the same time as baking inside the oven.
4. Another option is to fry the rice in a pan. Heat a small amount of olive or coconut oil in a frying pan over medium heat. Add the cauliflower rice to the pan and stir-fry the rice for 5 minutes. Serve the rice warm with finely chopped spring onion.

NUTRITIONAL VALUES

Serving size: 100 gr
Calories: 24

Fats: 0
Carbohydrates: 3.0

Proteins: 2.0

Balsamic mushrooms

Cooking time: 10 mins   **Total time: 15 mins**

INGREDIENTS

- 45 ml olive oil
- 3 cloves of garlic, finely chopped
- 450 gr fresh mushrooms
- 45 ml balsamic vinegar
- 45 ml of white wine
- salt and pepper to taste
- dried parsley to taste

PREPARATION METHOD

1. Saute the garlic in olive oil for 1 to two minutes. Add the mushrooms and fry for any other 2 mins, stirring once in a while inside the skillet. Then upload the balsamic vinegar and white wine and fry for another 2 mins. Season the mushrooms with salt and pepper.

NUTRITIONAL VALUES

Serving Size: ¼   Fats: 10.8
Calories: 126   Carbohydrates: 2.3Proteins: 2.9

Mushroom pizza

Cooking time: 15 mins   **Total time: 25 mins**

INGREDIENTS

- 2 XXL mushrooms (portobello)
- 30 ml pasta sauce
- 75 gr grated mozzarella

- 6 slices of spicy salami
- 2 black olives, cut into pieces
- 1 clove of garlic, finely crushed

PREPARATION METHOD

1. Preheat the oven to 190 degree. Remove the stem from the mushroom and region the XXL mushroom 'hat' on a baking tray, and bake the mushroom for 5 minutes in the preheated oven.
2. Remove the mushroom from the oven after baking and spread the pasta sauce over the mushroom. Then positioned the mozzarella, olives, salami, and garlic on the sauce's pinnacle. Bake the mushroom for every other 15-20 mins inside the preheated oven.

NUTRITIONAL VALUES

Serving Size: 1 mushroom pizza   Fat: 16.7   Proteins: 17.7

Calories: 252   Carbohydrates: 6.7

Asparagus with Parmesan cheese

Cooking time: 15 mins

Total time: 25 mins

INGREDIENTS

- 500 gr green asparagus
- 40 gr grated Parmesan cheese
- 15 ml of olive oil
- salt and pepper to taste
- optional: 40 ml balsamic vinegar

PREPARATION METHOD

1. Preheat the oven to 230 degrees. Place the asparagus on a baking tray and drizzle with olive oil. Then divide and sprinkle the Parmesan cheese over the asparagus and season with freshly ground black pepper.
2. Bake the asparagus inside the preheated oven for 12 to fifteen minutes, till the cheese has melted and the asparagus is smooth, however still crispy. Serve straight away on warm plates and season the asparagus with balsamic vinegar if essential.

NUTRITIONAL VALUES

Serving Size: ¼

Fats: 5.1

Proteins: 5.3

Calories: 93

Carbohydrates: 7.0

Green beans with walnuts

Cooking time: 20 mins　　　　　　　　**Total time: 30 mins**

INGREDIENTS

- 500 gr green beans
- 60 gr walnuts
- 15 gr butter

- 15 ml of olive oil
- 1 tbsp parsley
- salt and pepper to taste

PREPARATION METHOD

1. Preheat the oven to one hundred seventy-five degree. Place the walnuts on a greased baking tray. Then placed the baking tray within the oven and baked the walnuts for 6-eight mins within the preheated oven.
2. Put the green beans in a pan of boiling water and upload salt to taste—Cook the green beans for approximately 5 mins. Then drain the beans and rinse with cold water.
3. Then melt butter and oil in a skillet over medium warmth. Add the green beans and fry for approximately four mins. Then upload the walnuts and parsley and season with salt and pepper.

NUTRITIONAL VALUES

Serving Size: 1 portion　　　　　　　　Carbohydrates: 8.1
Calories: 189　　　　　　　　　　　　　Proteins: 5.4
Fats: 14.2

Broccoli in almond-lemon butter

Cooking time: 5 mins

Total time: 15 mins

INGREDIENTS

- 1 large broccoli, cut into florets
- 60 gr butter
- 2 tsp lemon juice

- 1 tsp lemon zest
- 30 g sliced almonds

PREPARATION METHOD

1. Boil the broccoli florets for about 4 to eight minutes, then drain the florets. Melt the butter in a saucepan over medium warmth. When the butter has melted, remove the pan from the heat and upload the lemon juice, lemon zest, and almonds. Stir this nicely together and pour it over the broccoli.

NUTRITIONAL VALUES

Serving Size: ¼

Calories: 174

Fats: 15.2

Carbohydrates: 7.0

Proteins: 3.7

Roasted Cauliflower

Cooking time: 25 mins   **Total time: 40 mins**

INGREDIENTS

- 1 large cauliflower, separated into florets
- 1 - 2 cloves of garlic, crushed
- 3 tbsp olive oil

- 25 gr grated Parmesan cheese
- 1 tbsp chopped fresh parsley
- salt and pepper to taste

PREPARATION METHOD

1. Preheat the oven to 220 degrees and grease a big baking dish with butter or oil. Place the olive oil and garlic in a big resealable bag or container.
2. Additionally, put the cauliflower within the bag and shake it well to mix the substances. The cauliflower florets within the oven dish and sprinkle with salt and pepper to taste.
3. Bake the cauliflower for 25 minutes inside the oven, stirring once in a while within the baking dish. Remove the baking dish from the oven after 25 mins and sprinkle the florets with Parmesan cheese and parsley. Serve the roasted cauliflower as a side dish with a chunk of meat or fish.

NUTRITIONAL VALUES

Serving Size: 1/6   Carbohydrates: 8.6
Calories: 118   Proteins: 4.7
Fat: 8.2

Broccoli with cheese sauce

Cooking time: 15 mins   **Total time: 20 mins**

INGREDIENTS

- 300 gr broccoli, fresh or frozen
- 55 gr grated cheddar cheese (or another cheese)
- 40 gr melted butter
- salt and pepper to taste

PREPARATION METHOD

1. Heat a pan with water over medium warmness. When the water is boiling, upload the broccoli florets to the pan. Cook the florets until soft and company, approximately 5 mins. After cooking, drain the water from the pan and spoon the broccoli florets into a microwave-secure dish.
2. Pour the melted butter over the broccoli and season with salt and pepper. Sprinkle the grated cheddar cheese over the broccoli florets and location in the microwave. Microwave the broccoli florets for about 1 minute until the cheese has melted.

NUTRITIONAL VALUES

Serving Size: ¼   Carbohydrates: 3.6
Calories: 152   Proteins: 5.6
Fat: 13.5

Green beans with bacon

Cooking time: 20 mins   **Total time: 30 mins**

INGREDIENTS

- 6 slices of baking bacon
- 55 gr sliced onions
- 1 - 2 cloves of garlic, finely chopped
- 300 gr fresh green beans, cleaned
- 160 ml of water
- salt and pepper to taste

PREPARATION METHOD

1. Place the bacon slices in a large and deep-frying pan. Fry over medium warm until fats come out of the bacon. Meanwhile, reduce the garlic into small pieces, clean the green beans, and take away the ends.
2. Then add the sliced onions and garlic to the pan and fry for 1 minute. After 1 minute, add the water and green beans to the frying pan. Let the beans boil until the water has evaporated and the green beans are gentle. If the green beans are not yet cooked, upload some greater water and await it to evaporate.
3. Add the pepper and salt and serve the dish in four quantities. The green beans with bacon may be served as a starter, but it's also scrumptious with the main course with a chunk of meat.

NUTRITIONAL VALUES

Serving Size: ¼   Fat: 5.4   Proteins: 6.2

Calories: 97   Carbohydrates: 7.0

Baked asparagus

Cooking time: 10 mins   **Total time: 15 mins**

INGREDIENTS

- 350 gr green asparagus
- 50 gr butter
- 2 tbsp olive oil

- 1/2 tsp salt
- 1/4 tsp ground black pepper
- 2 - 3 cloves of garlic, crushed

PREPARATION METHOD

1. Clean the asparagus and reduce a small piece of each stem's lowest. Heat the butter in a frying pan over medium heat. Add the olive oil and fry it briefly. Then add the pressed garlic, salt, and pepper and fry it for 1 minute within the butter and oil.
2. Then upload the asparagus and fry it for 10 minutes, turning the asparagus on occasion to ensure that they are all cooked equally. Serve the fried asparagus with a bit of meat or fish.

NUTRITIONAL VALUES

Serving size: 1/3 of the total
Calories: 200
Fats: 19.8

Carbohydrates: 3.6
Proteins: 1.2

DESSERT AND SNACKS

Low-carb New York cheesecake

Cooking time: 20 mins
Total time: 80 mins

INGREDIENTS

- Bottom
- 150 gr almond flour
- 25 gr coconut flour
- 75 gr butter, melted
- 30 g erythritol
- 1/4 tsp salt
- Stuffing
- 225 gr mascarpone
- 250 gr cream cheese
- 40 gr erythritol
- 3 eggs (M)
- 1 tsp vanilla extract
- 15 gr Steviala Sweet & Vanilla
- optional: 3 g gelatin powder

PREPARATION METHOD

1. Preheat the convection oven to one hundred seventy degree. Add all the backside substances to a mixing bowl and mix or knead into a smooth batter. Cover a cake tin or springform pan (24 cm) with a baking paper sheet.

2. Bake the bottom for approx.—15 to twenty minutes inside the preheated oven. The bottom is prepared whilst it has a pleasing golden-brown shade. Let the lowest cool out of doors the oven.

3. Now lower the oven temperature to 150 degrees. Grab a huge bowl and upload all of the ingredients for the filling. Then beat this for approx. 2 mins with an electric mixer till creamy. Then divide the filling over the cooled bottom.

4. Place an oven dish or baking tray filled with two hundred ml of water at the bottom of the oven. Now vicinity the spring shape in the oven's middle on a rack. Bake the cheesecake for 60 mins inside the preheated oven (150 degree).

5. When the cheesecake is ready, turn off the oven and go away the oven door ajar. Let the cheesecake cool to room temperature, after which positioned inside the fridge for approximately 4 to six hours. Or preferably the entire nighttime. Cut .. Into pieces and experience!

NUTRITIONAL VALUES

Serving Size: 1 slice (1/12)   Fat: 24.9   Proteins: 6.5
Calories: 264   Carbohydrates: 2.3

Low-carbohydrate cake roll with strawberries

12.

Cooking time: 50 mins

Total time: 65 mins

INGREDIENTS

- Cake roll
- 4 eggs (M)
- 60 gr almond flour
- 20 gr erythritol
- 4 grams of baking powder
- 1 tsp vanilla extract
- Strawberry jelly
- 200 gr strawberries
- 2 tbsp water
- 1/4 tsp lemon juice

- 10 g erythritol
- 1 gelatin sheet
- Whipped cream filling

- 150 gr whipped cream
- 100 gr MonChou cream cheese
- 20 gr erythritol
- Topping (optional)
- 50 gr sugar-free white chocolate
- 50 gr sugar-free milk chocolate
- 1/2 tsp vanilla extract

PREPARATION METHOD.

1. Strawberry jam. Soak the gelatin sheet in cold water for 10 mins. Then upload the strawberries, water, lemon juice, and erythritol to a saucepan. Put this at the hearth and allow it to boil for about five minutes, even as stirring. Then squeeze out the gelatin sheet and upload it simultaneously as stirring until it has melted. Then use a fork to press the strawberries to the favored thickness. Spoon the strawberry jam into a bowl and allow it to cool down.

2. Cake roll. Preheat the convection oven to 180 degree. Then you put a baking tray (forty × 40 cm) equipped with a bit of baking paper. Split 2 eggs. Then upload the egg whites with the erythritol to a big mixing bowl. Beat the egg whites with an electric mixer and set them apart.

3. Now take a brand new bowl and add the final 2 eggs, egg yolks, vanilla extract, almond flour, and baking powder. Mix this with a whisk to a smooth batter. Then spatula lightly through the egg whites. Spoon the batter onto the baking paper. Spread this out lightly, approximately 1 cm thick, and bake for 12 minutes within the preheated oven.

4. Whipped cream filling. Prepare the whipped cream filling while baking. To do this, upload the whipped cream, monchou cream cheese, and erythritol to a bowl and beat with an electric mixer until creamy.

5. Cake roll. Remove the cake from the oven after baking. Place a bit of parchment paper on your counter. Now take the cake and flip it over on a baking paper sheet. Remove the top sheet, cover the cake with the strawberry jam, and then the whipped cream filling. Now roll the cake tightly together with your palms and wrap the roll with household pores and skin foil. Place inside the fridge and permit it set for a minimum of 30 minutes.

6. Topping. Melt the chocolate au-bain-marie in a heat-resistant bowl over a saucepan with water. Divide the chocolate over the cake roll with a spoon. Cut the cake roll into approx. 13 slices. Store the cake roll within the fridge or keep with the slice within the freezer. Enjoy your meal!

NUTRITIONAL VALUES

Serving Size: 1 slice (1/13) without chocolate

Calories: 114
Fats: 10.1

Carbohydrates: 1.6
Proteins: 3.5

White chocolate mousse with raspberries

Cooking time: 10 mins
Total time: 90 mins

INGREDIENTS

- Mousse
- 125 ml of whipped cream
- 1 egg (m)
- 1/2 sheet of gelatin
- 30 g erythritol
- 75 gr white chocolate , sugar free
- Raspberry jelly:
- 100 gr raspberries
- 1/2 sheet of gelatin
- 20 gr erythritol

Topping

- raspberries as desired
- blueberries as desired
- grated white chocolate

PREPARATION METHOD.

1. Please start with the raspberry jelly to chill in the mousse's preparation course. Soak the gelatin in cold water and add the raspberries and erythritol to a saucepan. Bring this to a boil.
2. Pour the boiling jelly through a sieve right into a box. Press the sieve nicely with a spoon to simplest the seeds remain. Add the gelatin to the jelly while stirring. Set the jelly aside and keep with the mousse
3. Also, for the mousse, soak the gelatin in cold water. Then beat the whipped cream with an electric-powered mixer in a large mixing bowl. Now take saucepans and position them at the fireplace with a water layer.
4. Place heat-resistant bowls on the pinnacle of the two saucepans. Add the white chocolate to at least one bowl and the egg and erythritol to the alternative. Melt the chocolate and beat the egg creamy and fluffy with a whisk. Then put off the dish with the egg from the saucepan and upload the gelatin simultaneously as stirring.
5. Now grasp an electric-powered mixer and maintain beating until the egg mixture is at room temperature. Then cautiously fold the melted white chocolate into the egg aggregate and, sooner or later, the whipped cream.
6. Spread some culmination and raspberry jelly on the lowest of the glasses. Then divide 1/2 of the white chocolate mousse over the four glasses. Add some raspberry jelly and the last chocolate mousse. Top it off with a layer of raspberry jelly and a few fruits.
7. Put the dishes within the fridge for at least 1 hour earlier than serving. The longer the mousse is within the refrigerator, the stiffer it turns into.

NUTRITIONAL VALUES

Serving Size: 1 bowl (1/4)   Fats: 18.6   Proteins: 3.5
Calories: 225   Carbohydrates: 4.9

Low-carbohydrate eton mess

Cooking time: 45 mins

Total time: 75 mins

INGREDIENTS

- meringues
- 2 proteins (M)
- 25 g erythritol
- pinch of salt
- Forest fruit sauce
- 40 gr strawberries
- 20 gr raspberries
- 15 ml of water
- 10 g erythritol

Stuffing

- 200 ml whipped cream, 35% fat
- 100 gr mascarpone
- 1 tsp vanilla extract
- 40 gr erythritol

Topping:

- 50 gr raspberries
- 60 gr strawberries
- 50 gr blueberries
- 50 gr blackberries
- optional: fresh mint

PREPARATION METHOD

1. Preheat the convection oven to 140 degree. Split the eggs and upload the egg whites together with the erythritol and a pinch of salt to a mixing bowl. Beat the egg whites with an electric mixer within approx. 3 mins.

2. Then scoop the beaten egg whites with a spoon onto a baking tray covered with parchment paper. Spread the egg whites to an excellent thickness and bake for forty-five minutes in the preheated oven. Let the froth settle down after baking.

3. Meanwhile, make the wooded area fruit sauce to add all of the substances for the sauce to a pan. Place the pan on medium warmth and produce the fruits to a boil. Let it simmer for 2 mins while stirring. Then flip off the heat and let it cool to room temperature. Use a hand blender to make a clean sauce from the result.

4. Now take a new bowl and add all of the filling ingredients. Beat the whole lot with an electric-powered mixer until mild and stiff. After beating, put the filling in the refrigerator.

5. Now fall apart the meringue and upload it to a bowl. Grab your dessert glasses and start constructing. Add a handful of meringues to the glass and placed a few fresh culmination on the pinnacle. Now add 2 tbsp whipped cream filling and a bit of the sauce. Repeat this till all of your elements are long past.

6. Decorate the glasses with clean mint is essential. Do no longer prepare the Eton mess until you serve it. The foam will become smooth in the fridge. Enjoy your meal!

NUTRITIONAL VALUES

Serving Size: 1 bowl (1/4)

Calories: 317

Fats: 30.2

Carbohydrates: 6.7

Proteins: 5.5

Low-carbohydrate mini tiramisu

Cooking time: 30 mins

Total time: 45 mins

INGREDIENTS

- Sponge base
- 35 gr almond flour
- 5 gr coconut flour
- 1/4 tsp baking powder
- 1 egg
- 1/2 tsp vanilla extract
- 1 tbsp whipped cream
- 25 g erythritol
- 50 gr ricotta
- 1 espresso

Stuffing

- 50 ml whipped cream
- 75 gr mascarpone
- 1 egg yolk
- 1/2 tsp vanilla extract
- 20 gr Steviala Frost
- cocoa powder to taste

PREPARATION method

1. Preheat the convection oven or air fryer to 175 degree. In a massive bowl, blend the almond flour, coconut flour, baking powder, and erythritol nicely collectively. Then upload the ricotta, whipped cream, vanilla extract, and egg to the bowl. Stir the contents of the bowl with a whisk till smooth.

2. Grease a large ramekin (12 cm) or small ramekins (7 cm) with a little butter or oil. Then divide the batter from the bowl flippantly between the two ramekins. Place the ramekins in the oven or air fryer and bake for approximately 20 minutes inside the air fryer or 25-30 minutes inside the oven. After 10 mins, cowl the ramekins with aluminum foil so that the pinnacle does now not turn brown.

3. Meanwhile, make the filling using whipping the whipped cream with an electric-powered mixer until stiff in a cold bowl. While beating, add the mascarpone, vanilla, erythritol, and egg yolk. Whisk until stiff peaks shape. Do not beat too lengthy, as this may create a better structure.

4. When the lowest has cooled, you may cautiously pour 1 brewed espresso over the two bottoms. Then spread the mascarpone filling over the bottoms and garnish with cocoa powder. Enjoy your meal!

NUTRITIONAL VALUES

Serving Size: 1 bowl

Calories: 450

Fats: 42.3

Carbohydrates: 4.7

Proteins: 12.8

Low-carbohydrate strawberry flan

Cooking time: 30 mins   **Total time: 110 mins**

INGREDIENTS

- Bottom
- 200 gr almond flour
- 20 gr coconut flour
- 1 egg (M)
- 110 gr butter, unsalted
- 40 gr erythritol
- pinch of salt
- Custard

- 200 gr whipped cream
- 40 gr erythritol
- 3 egg yolks
- 1 tsp vanilla extract
- 2 gr gelatin powder

Topping
- 200 gr whipped cream
- 75 gr mascarpone

- 40 gr erythritol
- 1/2 tsp vanilla extract
- 300 gr strawberries
- optional: mint
- optional: almond flakes

PREPARATION METHOD.

1. Preheat the convection oven to 175 degree. In a massive bowl, combine all of the elements for the base. Then mix everything nicely along with your palms to shape a dough ball—grease a cake tin (25 cm) with butter, or line the tin with baking paper.
2. Divide the dough over the cake tin and make a raised facet. Then bake the bottom within the preheated oven for 25-30 minutes, until it's miles golden brown. Allow the lowest to cool completely after baking.
3. Meanwhile, make the pastry cream to add the egg yolks to a bowl at the side of a dash of whipped cream. Beat the yolks and set them aside. Then heat the last whipped cream in a small saucepan. When it's far heat, add the gelatin, vanilla, and erythritol whilst stirring, till the entirety is dissolved.
4. Now add the egg yolks with cream. Heat the pan's contents, even as stirring, until the cream has thickened. Turn off the heat and allow the pastry cream to cool to room temperature. Then add the cream to the cooled bottom and put it inside the fridge for approximately 1 hour.
5. Meanwhile, make the whipped cream topping using whipping cream, mascarpone, erythritol, and vanilla in a bowl until stiff. Remove the cake from the refrigerator and use a spatula to unfold the topping over the cake. Decorate the cake with strawberries and probably mint and almond shavings. Enjoy your meal!

NUTRITIONAL VALUES

Serving Size: 1 slice (1/12)   Fat: 28.2   Proteins: 6.8

Calories: 337   Carbohydrates: 4.3

Low-carbohydrate white chocolate cheesecake

Cooking time: 10 mins

Total time: 300 mins

INGREDIENTS

- Bottom
- 100 gr almond flour
- 60 gr melted butter
- 40 gr erythritol
- 1 egg yolk
- 2 tsp cinnamon
- 1 tsp gingerbread spices

Stuffing
- 225 gr mascarpone
- 200 ml whipped cream
- 150 gr monchou
- 150 gr white chocolate , sugar free
- 40 gr erythritol

- 15 gr gelatin powder

Topping
- 150 gr raspberries
- 3 tbsp water
- 5 gr gelatin powder
- optional: white chocolate
- optional: fresh fruit

PREPARATION METHOD

1. Preheat the convection oven to a hundred and seventy degrees. Then mix all of the bottom elements nicely in a large bowl. Line a springform pan (sixteen cm) with baking paper, both the bottom and aspects. Pour the batter into the tin and bake the lowest in the oven for about 30 minutes.
2. Meanwhile, in a huge bowl, beat the monchou and mascarpone fluffy with an electric mixer. Add the erythritol while mixing. Now take another bowl and whip one hundred fifty ml creamy cream in it until it has doubled in extent. Add the whipped cream to the monchou and mascarpone and whisk collectively.
3. Fill a saucepan with a layer of water. Bring the water to a boil and area a warmth-resistant bowl on the pan. Put the white chocolate in the bowl and melt the chocolate au-bain-marie. After melting, progressively stir the chocolate into the monchou mixture.
4. Meanwhile, warm the final 50 ml of whipped cream in a small pan. Add 15 grams of gelatin powder to the recent whipped cream whilst stirring. Be careful now not to permit the whipped cream to boil. Add the whipped cream with dissolved gelatin to the monchou combinations simultaneously as stirring.
5. Pour the monchou mixture into the spring shape with the cooled bottom and permit the cheesecake to set in the fridge for a minimum of three hours.
6. Start with the topping after 3 hours. To do that, puree the raspberries and add them to a saucepan. Add three tbsp water and switch on the warmth. Heat the raspberries over low heat and when the mixture is warm, add five g gelatin powder. Melt the powder and flip off the warmth.
7. Remove the cake from the refrigerator and pour the topping over it. Let the cake stiffen for another 2 hours, beautifying with white chocolate and sparkling fruit if necessary. Enjoy your meal!

NUTRITIONAL VALUES

Serving Size: 1 slice (1/12)

Fats: 30.1

Proteins: 4.7

Calories: 320

Carbohydrates: 4.0

Low-carbohydrate coconut pudding

Cooking time: 10 mins
Total time: 135 mins

INGREDIENTS

- 50 gr grated coconut
- 20 gr Steviala Crystal
- 50 gr cream cheese or dairy spread
- 1 egg, beaten
- 125 ml of whipped cream
- 150 ml coconut milk
- 1 tsp vanilla aroma

PREPARATION METHOD

1. In a microwave-safe bowl, mix 1/2 of the whipped cream with the grated coconut, Steviala Kristal, and vanilla aroma. Microwave the bowl (700 Watt) for a minute and set aside. If you do not have a microwave, you can also heat it short in a saucepan. In the meantime, beat the egg in some other bowl and upload the remaining whipped cream.
2. Now warmth the coconut milk and cream cheese in a saucepan till the cream cheese has melted. Then add the whipped cream with grated coconut to the pan. Heat this in short, and sooner or later, add the crushed egg with the whipped cream. Heat this whilst stirring until the pudding begins to thicken. Turn off the heat when the combination starts evolved to boil.
3. Pour the mixture into 4 small ramekins or dessert glasses and allow it to set within the fridge for at least 2 hours. Garnish the coconut pudding with a bit of grated coconut earlier than serving. Enjoy your meal!

NUTRITIONAL VALUES

Serving Size: 1 bowl
Calories: 300

Fat: 29.5
Carbohydrates: 3.6

Fiber: 2.3
Proteins: 4.1

Low-carbohydrate chocolate mousse

Cooking time: 15 mins
Total time: 135 mins

INGREDIENTS

- 250 ml of whipped cream
- 150 gr dark chocolate, 85% cocoa
- 40 - 50 g erythritol
- 3 medium eggs
- 1 tsp vanilla aroma
- pinch of salt

PREPARATION METHOD

1. Pour the whipped cream right into a big bowl. Make certain the whipped cream and bowl are cold. Beat the whipped cream with an electric-powered mixer at a medium pace and on the quit at an excessive velocity. Beat till peaks begin to shape. Do not beat too lengthy, due to the fact then a type of butter may additionally form and that is irreversible. Put the whipped cream inside the fridge after whipping

2. Fill a saucepan with a layer of water and produce it to a boil. Then place a heat-resistant bowl on the pinnacle of the saucepan and soften the dark chocolate in a bain-marie. After melting, permit the chocolate relaxation at room temperature.

3. Now get an easy heatproof bowl and add the eggs, erythritol, and salt to the bowl. Place the bowl on top of the saucepan with the boiling water, taking care not to allow the water to touch the bowl. Beat with the mixer on the very best setting, till the egg combination feels lukewarm. Then do away with the bowl from the pan and hold whisking on the counter till the aggregate has cooled down.

4. Add the melted chocolate alongside the vanilla aroma to the egg mixture and beat it properly. Finally, gently fold the whipped cream into the chocolate mixture till nicely mixed. Spoon the low-carb chocolate mousse into 6 small dessert glasses, cover with cling movie and allow it set in the fridge for at least 2 hours. Enjoy your meal!

NUTRITIONAL VALUES

Serving Size: 1 small dessert glass
Calories: 317

Fats: 29.3
Carbohydrates: 5.2

Proteins: 6.3

Lemon panna cotta

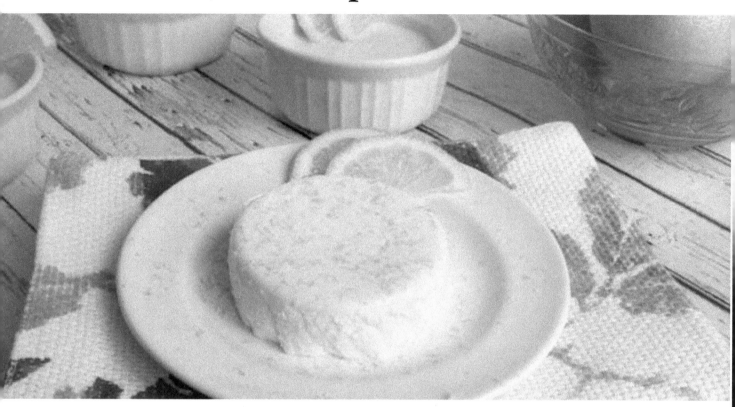

Cooking time: 5 mins   **Total time: 185 mins**

INGREDIENTS

- 250 ml of whipped cream
- 125 gr Greek yogurt
- 3 gelatin sheets
- 30 gr Steviala Crystal
- juice of 1 lemon
- 1 tsp grated lemon zest

PREPARATION METHOD

1. Heat the whipped cream in a pan with the steviala. Soak the gelatine sheets in cold water for 5 minutes. Squeeze the gelatin leaves and add them to the whipped cream inside the pan
2. Stir till the gelatin leaves dissolve, but don't allow it to boil. Then upload the yogurt and lemon juice whilst stirring. Mix till clean, after which eliminate the pan from the warmth.
3. Divide the cream mixture among four big or 6 small dessert glasses. Let them set in the refrigerator for at least 4 hours. Before serving, garnish the panna cotta with grated lemon zest and a lemon wedge. Enjoy your meal!

NUTRITIONAL VALUES

Serving Size: 1 bowl   Fat: 15.6   Proteins: 1.6

Calories: 156   Carbohydrates: 2.2

Low-carbohydrate almond magnums

Cooking time: 10 mins
Total time: 180 mins

INGREDIENTS

- 200 ml whipped cream
- 50 gr peanut butter
- 85 gr dark chocolate, 85% cocoa
- 1 vanilla pod
- 25 gr Steviala Crystal
- 60 ml almond milk
- 20 g almonds, chopped into pieces

PREPARATION method

1. Take a huge bowl and beat the whipped cream with an electric mixer until stiff. When the whipped cream is almost set, upload the Steviala crystal. Then upload the peanut butter and almond milk and gently stir it into the whipped cream.
2. Then region the vanilla pod on a reducing slice or plate and cut the stick open lengthwise with a pointy knife. Then spread the stick. You can see all varieties of small black seeds inside the stick. Now take a small spoon or a stupid knife and scrape out the vanilla pith (the small black seeds) and add it to the whipped cream.
3. Stir the entirety collectively nicely and divide the whipped cream mixture over 4-6 ice cream molds, depending on your molds' size. Put a stick in the ice creams and place it within the freezer for at least 3 hours.
4. Melt the chocolate au-bain, Marie, while the ice lotions are tough. When the chocolate has melted, eliminate the ice lotions from the molds. You can try this by strolling a few cold glasses of water over the molds. Place the finely chopped almonds on a plate. Then dip the ice lotions in the chocolate and then inside the finely chopped almonds. Let it harden inside the freezer and experience!

NUTRITIONAL VALUES

Serving size: 1 magnum   Fat: 23.5   Proteins: 4.1
Calories: 254   Carbohydrates: 3.3

Mascarpone dessert with berries

Cooking time: 10 mins   **Total time: 10 mins**

INGREDIENTS

- 115 gr mascarpone
- 125 ml of whipped cream
- 3 tbsp Steviala Kristal or to taste
- 250 gr strawberries
- 125 gr blueberries

PREPARATION METHOD

1. In a large bowl with an electric mixer, beat the mascarpone, whipped cream, and Steviala crystal together on the highest setting till stiff peaks form.
2. Cut the strawberries into small cubes and divide them between your six maximum lovely dessert glasses. Then divide the mascarpone over the glasses and top it off with the blueberries. Enjoy your meal!

NUTRITIONAL VALUES

Serving size: 1 glass   Fats: 15.2   Proteins: 1.8
Calories: 169   Carbohydrates: 5.4

Meringue

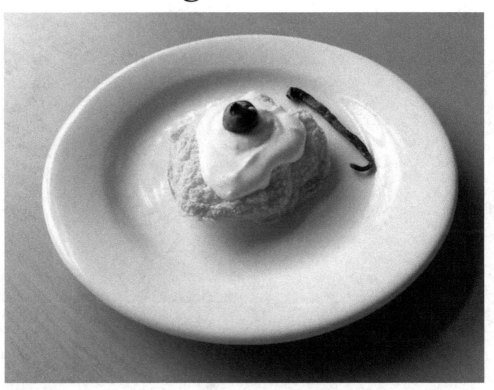

Cooking time: 20 mins
Total time: 40 mins

INGREDIENTS

- proteins from 4 medium eggs
- Steviala crystal to taste
- few drops of lemon aroma
- 100 gr mascarpone
- 100 ml of whipped cream
- 1/2 vanilla pod or vanilla aroma
- handful of fruit

PREPARATION METHOD

1. Preheat the oven to one hundred fifty degree. Then take a massive bowl and beat the egg whites, lemon flavor, and sweetener until stiff until peaks shape. Using a serving spoon, the crushed egg whites in hundreds on a baking tin included baking paper. Then push dimples inside the mounds and bake the pastries for forty mins inside the preheated oven.
2. Then cut the vanilla pod in half lengthwise. Use the stick's give-up as a deal with, and from there, pull a knife straight via the fruit. Use the blunt aspect of your knife to take the seeds out of the stick in one cross, urgent firmly, however no longer too difficult.
3. Take a bowl and mix the mascarpone, sweetener, and vanilla nicely collectively and set it apart. Now take another big bowl and beat the whipped cream in it. Fold the whipped cream into the mascarpone. Then take the meringues out of the oven after forty minutes and allow them to cool down. After cooling, divide the sauce over the meringues and serve with a few fruits.

NUTRITIONAL VALUES

Serving Size: 1/7   Fats: 10.8   Proteins: 3.1
Calories: 110   Carbohydrates: 1.2

Vanilla coconut ice cream

Cooking time:
240 mins
Total time: 240 mins

INGREDIENTS

- 2 cans of full-fat coconut milk
- 1 tsp vanilla aroma
- erythritol or stevia to taste

PREPARATION METHOD

1. Let the cans of coconut milk stiffen in the fridge for four hours. After 4 hours, remove the cans from the fridge. Remove the lid and let the remaining liquid in the cans drain.
2. Then put the remaining coconut fat collectively with the sweetener and vanilla aroma in a blender and blend till smooth. Put the combination in a plastic container and area the box within the freezer.
3. After 45 mins, cast off the box from the freezer, stirring the combination nicely once more. The stirring ensures that it remains a thick and creamy mixture. Repeat this until the container has been within the freezer for 4 hours.

NUTRITIONAL VALUES

Serving Size: 1/5   Fats: 24.2   Proteins: 3.2
Calories: 252   Carbohydrates: 2.5

Avocado chocolate cookies

Cooking time: 10 mins   **Total time: 20 mins**

INGREDIENTS

- 3 ripe avocados
- 30 gr protein powder (chocolate flavor)
- 140 gr almond flour
- 45 gr finely ground linseed

- 5 tbsp unsweetened cocoa powder
- 70 g sugar-free chocolate, chopped into pieces
- 1 medium egg

- 1 tsp baking powder
- 3 tbsp Steviala crystal

PREPARATION METHOD

1. Preheat the oven to 180 ranges. In a bowl, mix the almond flour, linseed flour, cocoa powder, stevia, egg white powder, and baking powder collectively. Then puree the avocado and stir it into the flour combination. Finally, upload an egg and blend properly.
2. Then stir the chocolate chips into the flour and avocado mixture. Shape the dough into 18 balls on the scale of your thumb. Then flatten the balls with a rolling pin.
3. Place the flat dough balls on a baking dish lined with baking paper. Bake the cookies in the oven for 10-12 mins. Then let them calm down for a while. Enjoy your meal!

NUTRITIONAL VALUES

Serving Size: 1 biscuit   Fat: 10.0   Proteins: 4.7
Calories: 143   Carbohydrates: 5.4

Strawberries dipped in chocolate

Cooking time: 5 mins   **Total time: 10 mins**

INGREDIENTS

- 100 gr dark chocolate (85%) or sugar-free chocolate
- 12 large strawberries
- optional: coconut grater or nuts

PREPARATION METHOD

1. Cover a baking tray with parchment paper. Cut the chocolate into small portions and region in a microwave secure bowl.
2. Place the chocolate in the microwave for 1 minute. Then put off the field from the microwave and stir the whole lot together properly. Then area the bowl inside the microwave for every other 20 seconds. Stir once more after 20 seconds and on the other hand in the microwave for 20 seconds. Repeat this manner till the chocolate has melted nicely. You can also melt the chocolate in a pan in a bain-marie (over boiling water).
3. When the chocolate has melted, put off the bowl from the microwave. Now dip thirds of each strawberry in the melted chocolate and optionally in the coconut grater or chopped nuts. Drain the strawberries over the bowl and then area them on the baking tray.
4. Then positioned the baking tray inside the refrigerator and permit the strawberries to cool for a half-hour.

NUTRITIONAL VALUES

S

erving Size: 4 strawberries   Fats: 3.0   Proteins: 0.5

Calories: 54   Carbohydrates: 5.2

Low-carbohydrate banana muffins

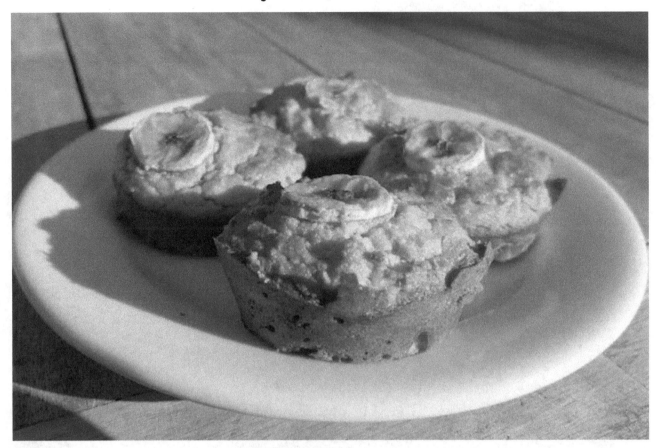

Cooking time: 15 mins   **Total time: 20 mins**

INGREDIENTS

- 200 gr almond flour
- 1 tsp baking powder
- pinch of salt

- 2 - 3 tbsp Steviala crystal
- 150 - 200 ml coconut milk

- butter for greasing
- 2 medium eggs
- 2 small ripe bananas

PREPARATION METHOD

1. Preheat the oven to a hundred and eighty degree. Then take a muffin tin for 12 portions and grease it with butter. Grab a blender and grind 1.5 bananas in it.
2. In a large bowl, combine the almond flour, baking powder, and salt. Then take some other bowl and beat together the eggs, coconut milk, finely ground banana, and Steviala crystal.
3. Carefully upload the egg aggregate to the flour and mix it. Divide the batter over the 12 ramekins and slice the last half banana. Garnish each muffin with a slice of banana. Bake the banana cakes for 20-25 mins in the preheated oven and experience!

NUTRITIONAL VALUES

Serving Size: 1 muffin   Fats: 12.0   Proteins: 4.7
Calories: 146   Carbohydrates: 6.4

Low-carbohydrate apple and cranberry cake

Cooking time: 45 mins   **Total time: 55 mins**

INGREDIENTS

- 3 - 4 medium eggs
- 350 gr applesauce, without added sugar
- 135 gr almond flour

- 2 tbsp coconut flour
- 45 gr vanilla protein powder
- 1 1/2 tsp baking powder

- 25 gr dried cranberries

PREPARATION METHOD

1. Preheat the oven to 175 degree. Then seize a bowl and blend within the eggs, baking powder, apple sauce, almond flour, protein powder, and coconut flour. Stir the contents with a whisk to a clean batter.

2. After stirring properly, upload the cranberries and stir them via the batter and set it apart. Now take a cake tin and grease it nicely with butter or oil. Pour the batter into the cake tin and unfold well. Bake the cake in the preheated oven till golden brown for about forty-five mins. After baking, allow it to cool down and cut into 14 slices.

NUTRITIONAL VALUES

Serving Size: 1 slice   Fat: 7.3   Proteins: 7.6

Calories: 120   Carbohydrates: 5.9

Low-carbohydrate cheesecake

Cooking time: 160 mins
Total time: 180 mins

INGREDIENTS

- Bottom:
- 175 gr almond flour
- pinch of salt
- 1 large egg
- 40 gr butter, melted
- 20 gr Steviala Crystal
- Cottage cheese filling:
- 500 gr low-fat cottage cheese
- 350 gr strawberries
- 250 ml of whipped cream
- 12 sheets of gelatin
- 100 ml of fresh orange juice
- 2 scoops of protein powder (vanilla or strawberry)
- dash of vanilla aroma

PREPARATION METHOD

1. Preheat the oven to a hundred and eighty degree. Take a massive bowl and blend the almond flour and salt with a whisk. Then add the big egg, Steviala Kristal, and the melted butter to the bowl and blend well. Take the cake tin and cover the lowest with baking paper. Press the dough onto the bottom of the pie crust and spread the dough frivolously. Bake the pie crust for 8 to 12 minutes inside the preheated oven.
2. Then take a bowl and fill it with cold water. Place the 12 gelatin sheets and let them soak for 5 minutes. Meanwhile, puree the 250 grams of strawberries in a blender. Put the one hundred ml sparkling orange juice in a saucepan and warm it over low heat. After 5 minutes soak, squeeze the gelatin leaves nicely. Remove the orange juice from the heat and mix inside the gelatin leaves even as stirring. Let the mixture cool.
3. In a massive bowl, stir together the low-fat quark, egg white powder, orange combination, and strawberry puree. In every other bowl, beat the whipped cream and vanilla aroma until stiff and scoop it lightly through the quark combination. Taste the aggregate and season with Steviala Kristal if vital. Divide the quark mixture over the almond base and permit it to set within the refrigerator for 3 hours.
4. After 3 hours, do away with the cheesecake from the refrigerator, reduce the final strawberries in half, and divide them over the low-carb cheesecake. Enjoy your meal!

NUTRITIONAL VALUES

Serving size: 1 slice

Calories: 330

Fats: 26.0

Carbohydrates: 9.5

Proteins: 17.3

Vanilla blueberry muffins

Cooking time: 20 mins   **Total time: 35 mins**

INGREDIENTS

- 5 medium eggs
- 1 tsp vanilla aroma
- 3 tbsp Steviala crystal
- 200 gr cream cheese
- 200 gr almond flour

- 1 tsp baking powder
- 30 gr butter
- 40 gr sugar-free chocolate
- 100 gr blueberries

- 1/2 tsp cinnamon
- pinch of salt

PREPARATION METHOD

1. Preheat the oven to 180 degree. Then mix the 5 eggs, 3 tbsp stevia, and 1 tsp vanilla aroma properly together in a bowl. Then add the 2 hundred grams of cream cheese to the bowl and mix until easy.
2. Then upload the almond flour, baking powder, cinnamon, butter, and a pinch of salt and beat till smooth. Pour the batter right into a greased muffin tray and divide the extra darkish chocolate and blueberries over the desserts. Bake the truffles for 20 to twenty-five minutes inside the preheated oven and allow them to quiet down after baking. Enjoy your meal!

NUTRITIONAL VALUES

Serving Size: 1 muffin   Fats: 14.2   Proteins: 6.7
Calories: 192   Carbohydrates: 3.4

Chocolate pecan pie

Cooking time: 30 mins
Total time: 50 mins

INGREDIENTS

Bottom:

- 260 gr almond flour, extra fine
- 2 tbsp coconut oil
- 1 medium egg
- 1/8 tsp salt
- 4 tbsp Steviala Kristal or to taste

Cake filling:

- 255 gr freshly grated zucchini or courgetti
- 130 g pecans, cut in half
- 85 g sugar-free extra dark chocolate
- 6 tbsp coconut oil, melted
- 3 medium eggs
- 1 1/2 tsp vanilla flavor
- 3 - 4 tbsp Steviala Kristal or to taste
- pinch of salt

PREPARATION METHOD

1. Preheat the oven to a hundred and eighty degree Celsius. Then grease a 23 cm cake pan with a touch of coconut oil. Make the bottom by mixing the almond flour, 2 tablespoons coconut oil, a pinch of salt, and 1 egg in a bowl. When properly blended, put the dough in the cake tin and lightly press the dough towards the lowest and area.
2. Now take the grated zucchini and squeeze the moisture out of the zucchini; you could do this via carefully squeezing the zucchini in a clean kitchen towel. Then put the grated zucchini, chocolate, melted coconut oil, vanilla extract, stevia, and the three eggs in a food processor and flip it on. Mix this for approximately 1 minute.
3. Then positioned the chocolate filling in a clean bowl and stirred in seventy-five% of the pecans. Then pour the chocolate pecan combination into the pie pan and sprinkle the ultimate pecans over the pie.
4. Bake the chocolate pecan pie for 30 to forty mins within the preheated oven. The cake is exceptional after cooling it in a single day within the refrigerator. Divide the cake into 12 quantities and revel in!

NUTRITIONAL VALUES

Serving size: 1 slice
Calories: 35
7Fat: 28.3

Carbohydrates: 3.2
Proteins: 4.5

CONCLUSION

Many people who hear the word ketosis for the first time look a little incredulous at first. What does it actually mean to follow a ketogenic diet and what are the benefits of the diet?

The keto diet is very popular with more and more people and numerous examples show that you can burn fatter if you turn the adjusting screws of your diet. Biohackers also use the ketogenic diet to increase their cognitive performance and keep the brain running at full speed.

The keto diet will help you burn excess body fat and have more energy. We'll show you what it means to eat a ketogenic diet.

Do you know the feeling when the scale suddenly shows a few kilograms more, even though you have not eaten too much? For people who are just about to lose some weight, the excess on the scales can be a real slap in the face. If you're one of those people who is desperately looking for a diet that works, you should give the ketogenic diet a try. Diet is based on healthy fats and high-quality proteins, while you cut down on carbohydrates and turn your body into a fat-burning machine.

There are many benefits to a ketogenic diet and it gets fat burning going. It also has a positive effect on mental and physical performance. However, some experts see the low vitamin intake in comparison to the high fat and protein intake over a longer period of time very critically.

Those who are aiming for weight loss can achieve good results with this diet. The keto diet, however, brings about a profound change in metabolism. This can lead to difficulties, especially in the initial phase. If you want to try the diet, you should always do so with professional or medical advice.